HEALTH AND FITNESS – OVER 50

Bob O'Connor & Christine Wells

The Crowood Press

First published in 1999 by
The Crowood Press Ltd
Ramsbury, Marlborough
Wiltshire SN8 2HR

British Library Cataloguing-in-Publication Data
A catalogue record for this book is available from the British Library.

ISBN 1 86126 208 6

Line-drawings by David Fisher.

Dedication
To Tyler James 'TJ' Wells, the light of our lives. While TJ has a bit more than 49 more years to reach the half-century mark, he gives us the best reason of all to continue in our healthy lifestyles so that we will be around to see him grow and mature. What better reason for living a vibrant middle age – with one eye on his future and the other on our own.

Acknowledgements
The authors would like to thank photographer Gerhard Pagels for his fine photographs and his attention to detail. We also thank our models from the Norwegian University of Sport and Physical Education: Professors Kari Fasting, Glyn Roberts, Marit Sørensen and Eystein Enoksen. And yes – they do practise what they preach. They all run, ski or cycle nearly every day.

Thanks also to the people at The Crowood Press who have been so professional in their approach to publishing and particularly to Ian Young, who had faith in the project, and Julie McRobbie, who saw it through.

Photographic Acknowledgements
Black and white photographs taken and/or supplied by the author, except where stated otherwise.

Typefaces used: Galliard and Franklin Gothic.

Typeset and designed by
D & N Publishing
Membury Business Park, Lambourn Woodlands
Hungerford, Berkshire.

Printed and bound in Great Britain by
J. W. Arrowsmith Ltd, Bristol.

Contents

Preface

First, a couple of truisms:

- People are living longer than ever before.
- The diseases of ageing are, to a large degree, environmental.
- We can live longer and better.

With these ideas in mind, many of us have decided to begin or to continue with fitness and nutritional habits which will make our lives fuller, our minds happier and our bodies younger. To become more effective in our lives we must first have goals. Once we have established our goals we must develop a plan, based on the best information of modern science, then stick to our plan. Unfortunately, many who begin new habits soon fall by the wayside. So we must have a firm commitment to live better – in both the physical and mental domains. When we do this, we can achieve unexpected rewards. As Henry David Thoreau has said, 'If one advances confidently in the direction of his dreams, and endeavours to live the life which he has imagined, he will meet with the success unexpected in common hours.'

If we are already practising good health habits we may want to apprise ourselves of the latest knowledge and perhaps add to or subtract from our current programme. If we are just beginning a programme we want our activities to be the most productive that they can be. We will want to fight through our cobweb-covered habits and make them into habits with the 'strength of cables' – to paraphrase an old Chinese proverb.

So let us look at the hurdles we face, our advancing age, the threats of heart disease and cancers, and the other attendant pitfalls, then see how we can overcome these obstacles with effective healthy behaviour. We *can* reverse many of the effects of advancing age and we *can* develop a greater joy in living. So why not?

ABOUT THIS BOOK

As we enter our mid-lives, we become increasingly aware that there are a number of things that we should do, and some things we should not do, in order to live longer and fuller lives. The aim of this book is to help you to develop a high level of personal health. It is fundamental to our lives. As the old Arabian proverb muses, 'He who has health has hope and he who has hope has everything.'

With our goal of vibrant physical and mental health in mind, we shall take a realistic look at the process and diseases of ageing, then look at what we can do about them based on the most recent research. We can definitely reduce our chances of developing heart disease, cancers and other illnesses. Our fate is not all hereditarily determined. We can exercise effectively to lengthen our lives and to avoid such problems of ageing as osteoporosis (soft bones). We can eat more effectively and we can also supplement our diet with vitamins and minerals which are now known to be needed. Contrary to some opinions, we cannot get enough of all of the necessary nutrients just by eating an ideal diet. We must supplement our diets.

Stress causes both physical and mental illness. We can learn to avoid stress and to cope with that stress which confronts us. It is not difficult to eat sensibly, to exercise effectively and to live happily. This book is designed to give you the *reasons why* and the *means to* live longer and more fully.

CHAPTER 1

Do You Honestly Want to Feel Better and Live Longer?

Anyone in his or her right mind wants to feel better and most of us would like to live longer – then why do so many of us continue the bad habits that make our lives shorter and less enjoyable? As has been said, 'He who has no time for his health today will have no health for his tomorrow.'

Scientists know that developing the right fitness and exercise habits can reduce our pot bellies, eliminate depression, make us proud of our bodies, give us more energy and reduce our chances of developing the diseases of ageing – such as diabetes, heart problems and high blood pressure, and even cancers.[1] We are all aware that a healthier regimen will enhance our lives. Then why don't we take the steps to do some or all of the things that science recognizes to be healthy?

We get into ruts – and you know a rut is a long grave! If we were fed fruit for dessert when we were young, we probably continue to eat fruit for dessert. If it was pastries and chocolate, we probably continue in that habit. If we exercised in our youth and enjoyed it, we are more likely to exercise today. But the ease of our twentieth-century lives makes it so easy to settle onto the couch, turn on the television, and take the easy path to killing time – and killing ourselves. If the only exercise you get is changing channels with the remote control, your thumb may be getting adequate exercise, but your heart is wasting away.

WHAT SHOULD BE OUR CONCERNS AS WE AGE?

Our quality of life must be considered both in health and in illness. That quality can be seen as both our objective functioning, how healthy or ill we really are, and by our subjective feelings about how and who we are. We may feel joy or pain, apprehension or certainty, depression or elation.[2] These feelings go a long way towards our determining that we are healthy. We must be positive about our chances for joy and longevity. More and more people are living to be 100 years old, and the number of centenarians is expected to quadruple within 20 years. Life seems to get better each year and more of us are interested in holding on to this good life.

If I want to live longer and better, I should be aware of what is happening as I age. We're not 20 anymore. At 20, our energy was generally high even without taking proper care of our bodies. As we age, we lose muscle tissue. We lose brain cells. Our body, at the level of our cells and tissues, does not function as efficiently as it once did. In fact, it seems that at about age 50 our degeneration begins to speed up.[3] So as we age it becomes imperative that we exercise and eat effectively in order to both slow our ageing and to reverse it.

If we are to be intelligent about changing our lives in a positive direction we should be aware of what is happening to us as we age. When we understand the ageing process we can avail ourselves of the programmes and products which science tells us will slow or reverse the processes of ageing. For this reason, in the next chapter we will look at some of the theories of how we age, then in the following chapter we will survey some of the diseases of ageing. After we have grasped the realities of what is, or may be, happening to us, we can more effectively plan on a fitness programme.

We would hope that as you see the potentials for living a longer and more fruitful life you will be more motivated to change your diet and exercise habits – if they need changing. We hope that we can also give you some ideas which may help to improve your mental health and to experience the happiness which results from such a positive change.

HOW CAN I CHANGE MY LIFE POSITIVELY?

You must decide that you *want* to make a permanent change. So many people start with good intentions. They give up smoking for a few weeks then go back to the weed. They start on a healthy diet then return to their deeply ingrained habits. They start to jog, get some muscle soreness, then retire to the sofa – watching other people exercise. Don't even start unless you want the change to be permanent. And if you choose to die earlier than necessary just consider that you are doing your bit to control world overpopulation!

Next, you will want to make your life changes as enjoyable as possible. You can watch the television while you ride your exercise bike, jump rope or walk on a home treadmill. If you don't want to change your diet to include all of the vitamins and minerals you need, you can pop some pills to give you these nutrients.

If you want to go to a gym, make it a social occasion – go with your friends every day or two. If you would rather garden or walk – no problem. Just make it enjoyable. Obviously a habit which makes you happy will be a great deal easier to learn than one that is drudgery or otherwise unpleasant.

Dr William Castelli, the director of the Framingham Heart Study – the longest on-going study in the world – became the first man in his family to live beyond 50 years of age. He did it by heeding his own advice of not smoking, restricting fat in his diet and exercising. At 60 he was as fit as a fiddle. You can add years to your life and life to your years – if you want to.

WHAT AND WHY DO YOU WANT TO CHANGE?

We will give you a number of reasons to make positive changes in your life. We will discuss diseases which can be avoided, or at least reduced, with proper health habits. We will give you a greater insight into why you should be more attentive to your diet, your exercise programme and your tobacco addiction. You choose which you want to change and how much.

Do you want to exercise just enough to live a bit longer or do you want to exercise to the point where your activity makes positive mental changes in your life? Do you want to lose weight in order to look and feel better, or to increase your longevity? Do you want to stop smoking for your own sake or for the sake of your family? We will lay out the facts – you decide if and what you want to do. It's your life!

We will start with the negatives – the diseases and negative health practices. Next we will look at improving your fitness by eating a more efficient diet, then we will look at various kinds of exercise programmes. We will try to make it as pleasant a change in your behaviour as possible. The rest is up to you!

MENTAL HEALTH

Our mental health is also often negatively affected as we age. We can be more adversely affected by the stresses of business, the changes in our family status and the obvious physical manifestations of the process of our getting older.

A book on fitness would not be complete without looking at our mental health and the opportunities to make it better – particularly through exercise.

A FINAL THOUGHT

The oft-quoted remark certainly seems to fit here – that the goal of life is to die young, as late as possible!

CHAPTER 2
Theories of How We Age

We know it's happening, but we don't know exactly why or how. If we did, we would be more able to slow the ageing process. But we *do* know some things and these things have helped many people to live longer and more effective lives. Better nutrition, especially eating less fat, and more exercise have allowed many of us to live longer than our parents and grandparents.

If we understand some of the theories of ageing that are being researched we can change our health behaviour to take advantage of what is known today. But we must remember that research into ageing does not have all of the answers. Our extremely complicated bodies with our own genetic predispositions and our varying environments give us trillions of variables for the researchers to investigate. We may never know all of the answers, but we do have some ideas.

If we ever completely understand how and why ageing occurs, the reasons will undoubtedly be a combination of the following theories plus some not yet postulated. The theories of ageing generally can be classified as 'built-in' or 'genetic', in which the cells break down, or they can be seen as 'damage' theories, in which the genetic material (DNA and RNA) is damaged so that it cannot function properly or reproduce healthy cells. Additionally, when we look at the following theories we can't be certain if ageing is a result or a cause of the factors which we observe.

While some wild optimists suggest, based on animal studies, that we might be able to live to be 200, we are a long way from such potential. But scientists around the world, such as those at the Department of Geriatric Medicine at the University of Manchester, are working to unlock the keys to living longer and better. And they are finding that we can each play a part in extending our own lives.

GENETIC THEORIES

Cell Doubling Theory

Cells of a species tend to multiply and reproduce themselves for a predetermined number of doublings. Once they have completed their predetermined number of doublings, the cell stops reproducing and the organism dies. It is assumed that the human being should be able to live between 110 and 120 years based on the number of doublings expected by human cells.

Studies with some non-human cells indicate that perhaps vitamin E can prolong the number of doublings. Other experiments have indicated that by lowering the body temperature the cells will double at a slower rate. If there were temperature-lowering drugs, life might therefore be lengthened.

The genetic switching theory holds that the genes have a built-in switch which begins ageing at a certain period of one's life. It is therefore similar to the 'cell doubling' theory.

The Error Catastrophe Theory

Deoxyribonucleic acid (DNA) and ribonucleic acid (RNA) are the basic genetic materials. DNA is the basic structure of the genes. It can reproduce itself with the help of the RNA. When either is changed, the gene cannot reproduce itself or cannot reproduce itself correctly.

This theory holds that the correct genetic information held in the DNA is changed by enzymes or the environment. This 'bad' information is then transmitted to other cells by the RNA. Damage could also have occurred to the RNA which would have resulted in its transmitting erroneous information.

Another theory suggests that the immune system which fights diseases reduces in efficiency as we become older. Problems such as cancers or illnesses therefore progress farther and faster as we age. Appropriate exercise can keep the immune system more efficient, as can a proper diet.

CELLULAR DAMAGE THEORIES

Free Radical Ageing Theory

In chemical reactions, both inside and outside of the body, non-stable atoms or molecules can be produced. Commonly oxygen, without one of its electrons (a free oxygen radical), attacks body cells in search of an electron which will make it stable. The action of the oxygen radical damages cells. When it attacks the collagen and elastin of the skin, wrinkles form. When it attacks the arteries in the heart, a lesion is formed which may then attract the cholesterol which narrows the arteries, setting up a heart attack. When it affects the tissues of the joints, arthritis can occur. When it attacks other areas of the body, cancers can begin. When it attacks brain tissues, dementia and Alzheimer's disease can be the result.

Free oxygen radicals are formed as part of the body's normal functioning, particularly when fats are oxidized in the body for energy. Their production is increased during exercise. Illness and stress also increase their production in the body. They are also present in, or are caused by, air pollution, water pollution, tobacco and other smoke, and sunlight.

A proper diet which is low in fats and high in antioxidants can reduce the risk of cell destruction. Reducing or controlling one's life stresses can also have a favourable effect on longevity. Obviously, smoke from tobacco, marijuana or any other source is also a negative environmental factor.

Toxic Waste Accumulation Theory

As we grow older, the reproduction of our cells and their ability to repair damage is reduced. This is caused by an accumulation of toxic wastes in the cells. These wastes often become free oxygen radicals which damage the cells. The sources of the wastes are both internal and external. The external sources include environmental pollutants such as pesticides, heavy metals and radiation. The internal sources are caused by oxidized fats such as overheated or rancid margarine, shortening, butter or liquid oils.

The Cross-Linkage Ageing Theory

Free radicals are again involved here. In this theory, they combine with proteins in such a way that the cells can no longer absorb nutrients, such as oxygen or water, from the blood. The connective tissues of the body, including collagen (the supporting protein of ligaments, skin and other tissues), become hardened, leading to stiffness in the tendons, wrinkled skin and cataracts in the lenses of the eyes. Along with the free oxygen radicals, sunlight, smog and stress can also cause cross-linking.

10

CHRONOLOGICAL AGE
AND BIOLOGICAL AGE

The number of years you have lived (chronological age) and the relative age of your body (biological age) are not the same. If your heredity has speeded up your ageing or if your environment has created more cell damage you will have a biological age which is older than your chronological age. If you have been stressed, have had excessive free oxygen radical damage because you have eaten too many fats, or if you have been exposed to smoke or other air pollution it is likely that your body is older than it should be.

A lack of exercise can also increase your biological age because the exercise you have not taken would have increased your immunity to diseases and would have kept your muscles and other organs healthier. It would have also reduced the chances of blood vessel damage through a build-up of cholesterol in the heart and brain. Similarly, if you had eaten wisely, minimized your fat intake and taken adequate antioxidant vitamins, your cells would have suffered less damage because they would have been exposed to fewer free oxygen radicals.

Biological ageing is, to a large degree, dependent upon the ability of your cells to repair themselves as quickly as they are damaged. When the damage occurs at a greater rate than your cells' ability to repair it, your biological age will increase.

PHYSICAL CHANGES OF AGEING

From the time we are 20 until the age of 75 we will lose:

- about 3in (7.6cm) in height;
- 10 per cent of our brain weight (primarily water);
- 30 per cent of our ability to pump blood from the heart (cardiac output);
- 65 per cent of our taste buds;
- 60 per cent of our ability to use oxygen (maximum oxygen uptake); and
- 20 per cent of our body's water content.

Additionally we may:

- become more sensitive to heat and cold;
- lose some bone (osteoporosis);
- develop kidney and bladder problems;
- become constipated more often due to the changes in the musculature of the large intestine;
- become more susceptible to medicines because the liver shrinks and the kidneys become less effective in eliminating wastes;
- lose some mental functioning due to the loss of brain neurons and the lessened ability of the neurotransmitters to work effectively.

SLOWING OR REVERSING
THE EFFECTS OF AGEING

It is estimated, based on studies involving twins, that about 20 per cent of our ageing and death potential is set in our genes. That means that about 80 per cent of our ageing and death factors are set by our environment – by where we live and how we live. We therefore have some power over our destinies.

When you understand the theories of ageing and the environmental contributions you make to your ageing through not exercising effectively, poor eating habits, smoking or drinking, and living a stressful life, you may decide to make some changes. If you will bear with us for one more chapter, that on disease, we will begin our exposé of those habits that contribute to our ageing and how we can change our ways.

There are a number of signs of ageing which become evident after age 25 or 30:

At age 40
- You use about 120 calories per day less than you did at 30, so weight control is more difficult.
- You will be about ⅗th of an inch shorter than at age 30 and you will continue to shrink about an inch every 15 years. This is due to bone loss, the compression of the spinal disks and changes in posture.
- A hearing loss will develop, particularly at the higher frequencies. Men have more problems with this than women.
- As the lenses of the eyes become harder there will be more difficulty in focusing on close things, such as newspaper print.

By the fifties
- Muscle cells atrophy and strength is lost.
- Immunity system continues to become less effective, increasing the chances of developing infections and cancers. This is due in part to the reduction in size of the thymus gland.
- The eyes become less sensitive to recognizing objects in dim light.

By the sixties
- The joints become stiffer due to less lubrication and the effects of 60 years of use.
- Men's sexual daydreams have pretty well stopped by the mid-sixties. The reason is unknown.
- Hearing continues to diminish.
- Diabetes increases as the functioning of the pancreas becomes less efficient.

By the seventies
- The harder artery walls make the heart pump harder so blood pressure increases, usually by 20 to 25 per cent.
- Coordination is reduced probably because of a diminished brain function.
- Short-term memory is reduced.
- Half of men show signs of coronary artery disease.
- Sweat glands become less efficient.

By the eighties
- Osteoporosis (loss of calcium in the bones) increases the risk of hip fracture and falling.
- Mental function continues to diminish with about 50 per cent of people showing signs of senility or Alzheimer's.

But as we look at each risk factor, we must bear in mind that no one is exactly average. While the average one pack a day smoker cuts his or her life span by seven years, there are those who smoke and live to be over 100. Of course, if we are looking at the averages, there must equally be a number of people shortening their lives by more than 7 years.

The importance of the risk factors is also something we may look at. While either not exercising or being obese is the number one factor, the third highest risk factor is either cholesterol levels or smoking. For the person who has hereditarily high cholesterol, such as

400 (the ideal being under 160 and the normal nearer 200), that person will probably not live to be 40, even following a healthy regimen. The high cholesterol level will become the primary risk factor. Your heredity is very important in determining just how negative each risk factor is for you. However, we must remember that the most important risk factors can generally be controlled by us (exercising effectively, being trim, having a low cholesterol level and not smoking) if we merely know where we stand in regard to each one.

For a person with very high cholesterol, only medication or an operation can help. Obesity

CALCULATE HOW LONG YOU WILL LIVE

This chart will give you a rough idea of how your life expectancy varies from the norm. To estimate how long you'll live, begin by using the table below to find the median life expectancy of your age group. Then add or subtract years based on the risk factors listed in the chart (you should adjust your risk-factor score by the percentages at right if you are over 60)

AGE	MALE	FEMALE	SCORING RISK FACTORS
20–59	73	80	use table as shown
60–69	76	81	reduce loss or gain by 20%
70–79	78	82	reduce loss or gain by 50%
80+	add five yrs to current age		reduce loss or gain by 75%

	Gain in life expectancy			*No change*	*Loss in life expectancy*			start with your median life expectancy
HEALTH	+3 YRS	+2YRS	+1YR		–1YR	–2YRS	–3YRS	TALLY
Blood pressure	Between 90/65 and 120/81	Less than 90/65 without heart disease	Between 121/82 and 129/85	130/86	Between 131/87 and 140/90	Between 141/91 and 150/95	More than 151/96	
Diabetes	–	–	–	None	Type II (adult onset)	–	Type I (juvenile onset)	
Total cholesterol	–	–	Less than 160	161–200	201–240	241–280	More than 280	
HDL cholesterol	–	–	More than 55	45–54	40–44	Less than 40	–	
Compared with that of others my age, my health is:	–	–	Excellent	Very good or fair	–	Poor	Extremely poor	
LIFESTYLE	+3 YRS	+2YRS	+1YR		–1YR	–2YRS	–3YRS	TALLY
Cigarette smoking	None	Ex-smoker, no cigarettes for more than 5 yrs	Ex-smoker, no cigarettes for 3–5 yrs	Ex-smoker, no cigarettes for 1–3 yrs	Ex-smoker, no cigarettes for 5 months –1 yr	Smoker, 0–20 pack-yrs*	Smoker, more than 20 pack-yrs	
Second-hand smoke exposure	–	–	–	None	0–1 hour per day	1–3 hours per day	More than 3 hours per day	
Exercise average (give yourself most positive category)	More than 90 min per day of exercise (e.g. walking) for more than 3 yrs	More than 60 min per day for more than 3 yrs	More than 20 min per day for more than 3 yrs	More than 10 min per day for more than 3 yrs	More than 5 min per day for more than 3 yrs	Less than 5 min per day	None	

CALCULATE HOW LONG YOU WILL LIVE (continued)

LIFESTYLE	+3 YRS	+2YRS	+1YR		−1YR	−2YRS	−3YRS	TALLY
Saturated fat in diet	–	Less than 6.7%	6.8%–14%	14.1%–19.3%	–	More than 19.3%	–	
Fruits and vegetables	–	–	5 servings per day	–	None	–	–	
FAMILY	**+3 YRS**	**+2YRS**	**+1YR**		**−1YR**	**−2YRS**	**−3YRS**	**TALLY**
Marital status	–	Happily married man	Happily married woman	Single woman, widowed man	Divorced man, widowed woman	Divorced woman	Single man	
Disruptive events in the past year†	–	–	–	–	One	Two	Three	
Social groups, friends seen more than once/month	–	Three	Two	One	–	None	–	
Parents' age of death	–	–	Both lived past 75	One lived past 75	–	–	Neither lived past 75	

* A pack-yr is one pack per day for a year. † Deaths of family members, job changes, moves etc.

your estimated life expectancy [ ]

Source: Michael F. Roizen, M.D., using data abstracted from the real age and age-reduction-planning programmes of medical informatics. *Newsweek* August 11, 1997.

In a large study of older and younger people in China it was concluded that there is a physiological basis for living longer. The major factors included:

- a better blood flow to the cells;
- a stronger, more efficient heart, lung and circulatory system;
- a more effective immune system;
- better adrenocortical, liver and kidney functions; and
- a higher level of high density lipoprotein cholesterol.

It was suggested that Chinese traditional medicine, along with Western medicine, might be used to improve the micro-bloodflow, nature killer cell activity, high density lipoprotein cholesterol and vital organ function.

(Department of Ageing and Anti-ageing, Shanghai Institute of Gerontology and Geriatrics, Huadong Hospital, People's Republic of China.)

may also need medical help – if it is hereditary. But smoking and exercise levels are definitely behaviours we can control without the help of others. If ageing is due to us taking poor care of our bodies, and there is growing evidence that it is, there is hope that solutions can be developed to slow the onset of the diseases of ageing. This will be a very difficult job.

The value of a genetic understanding of ageing is clear, but interventions need not be genetic. For example, regular athletic exercise is associated with a slowing of the accumulation of mutant mitochondria seen in muscle cells with advancing age. Exercise also reduces blood pressure and excess weight and changes the more dangerous cholesterols to the protective ones.

In ancient Rome, the average lifespan was about 22 years, now it is approaching eighty. In 1850, only one out of six Englishmen lived to be 75, today it is four out of six.[1] We must be doing some things right! The picture we now need to define is of how genes, environments and lifestyles work together to influence longevity and health in old age. This will not come easily, but come it will if we go at it hard enough. Increasing human life spans to 200 years may take a little longer.

At this point, it should be said, loudly and clearly, that the primary goal of research into the biological basis of ageing must be to increase the quality of the later years of life. If quality is not improved, any increase in longevity would not be a victory. Now let us first take a look at the diseases which are most likely to 'get us' then we can understand better what we need to do to live longer and better. Later, we will look at the mental side of our lives and suggest some ways to make our lives more fulfiling as we are living longer.

CHAPTER 3

The Diseases of the Blood Vessels

Most of the diseases which kill us are diseases to which we have contributed. We may neglect to have a physical examination which might detect an abnormality. We eat too much or exercise too little. Perhaps by understanding a bit more about how these diseases develop, we may decide to change our habits so that we can minimize our chances of developing the problem.

Most people die of diseases which are labelled as chronic or degenerative rather than those which are communicable. Five of the top ten causes of death are of the chronic-degenerative type which attack us as we age.

The ten top killers are:

1. Diseases of the heart
2. Cancer
3. Stroke (cerebral vascular accidents)
4. Bronchitis, emphysema, asthma
5. Accidents
6. Influenza and pneumonia
7. Diabetes
8. AIDS
9. Suicide
10. Homicide

The top four and the seventh are in the chronic and degenerative category. Other degenerative diseases are hardened arteries (atherosclerosis), arthritis, headaches, emphysema, multiple sclerosis, Alzheimer's disease and low back pain. These diseases can be inherited or developed by the way we live. A recent 21-year study in Scotland indicated that even our social class affects our chances of developing diseases and dying earlier. The men in the manual trades, and presumably lower social class, died at a higher rate than those who worked in the non-manual areas.[1]

CARDIOVASCULAR DISEASES

The major killer in the Western world is the combination of cardiovascular problems, affecting the heart and the blood vessels of the body. Coronary artery disease, a hardening of the blood vessels which supply blood to the heart, is the most frequent killer among the cardiovascular ailments. Stroke (cerebral vascular accident or CVA), a deadening of brain tissue, is also a blood vessel problem. In a recent study of male mortality in a number of European countries during the decade of 1980 to 1990, it was found that heart disease was greatly related to manual labouring people in England, Wales, Ireland, and the Scandinavian countries, but not in Switzerland, France or the Mediterranean countries; here, a number of cancers were a primary cause of death.[2]

The causes of heart attack and stroke are similar because in both cases the blood flow to the organ is slowed or stopped, resulting in a lack of oxygen and nutrients that deadens the heart muscle or brain tissue. The causes of

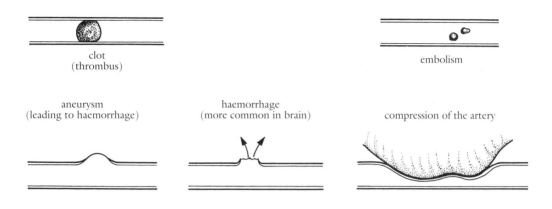

Fig 1. These four problems lead to most cardiovascular accidents. Obstructed blood vessels add more complications.

blood blockage can be a thrombus, a haemorrhage or compression.

The blood flow may be slowed or stopped by a thrombus, a clot which clogs the blood vessel. It may be slowed by an embolism. This moving clot can slow the blood flow so that the necessary oxygen does not reach the tissues ahead of the embolism. Blood flow can be slowed if the artery is constricted. This can happen if a growing tumour pushes down on the blood vessel. Or blood flow can be slowed if the artery ruptures and the blood haemorrhages.

Heart Attack

This is the most common type of heart ailment. It occurs when an artery of the heart is blocked. The coronary artery or the 'crowning' artery is the major artery of the heart, bringing blood to the heart muscle. Without that blood, the heart muscle will not have the oxygen that is needed and will cramp. This cramping is called a heart attack. The cramping of the muscle occurs in the area forward of the blockage. The area damaged during a heart attack can be so small

that the individual does not even know that a heart attack has occurred, or it can be so massive that the individual dies immediately.

When the heart attack occurs, there is a scarring of the heart muscle, causing the muscle's death. This is called a myocardial infarction, Latin for 'the death of the heart muscle'.

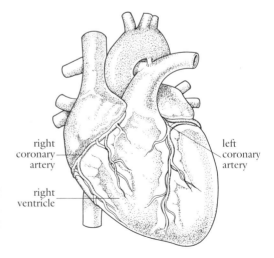

Fig 2. The healthy heart.

It used to be thought that the scarring was complete as soon as the heart attack had finished, but it is now known that there tends to be a continual scarring and it can spread. This is another reason for immediate expert attention, because effective doctors can minimize the damage that may continue after the first part of the heart attack.

Symptoms of Heart Attack

- An uncomfortable feeling of pressure, fullness or squeezing in the chest.
- Possible pain in the shoulder, arm, neck, lower jaw.
- Possible dizziness, fainting, nausea, shortness of breath.

If any of these symptoms last for more than a few minutes, call a doctor.

Each year, millions of people die from heart disease. Of these, 65 per cent of the people with severe coronary attacks die before reaching the hospital. But in three out of five cases people survive their first heart attack. Men are more likely to experience these than women, but after the menopause a woman's chances greatly increase and her risk is four times what it was before the menopause.

Strokes

These are the third leading cause of death, accounting for nearly 7 per cent of all deaths. But in people over 70, at least two out of every three deaths are from stroke. Men are more commonly afflicted than women.

A stroke occurs when a blood vessel in the brain is blocked or bursts and the oxygen supply to the brain is cut off. Since the brain requires about 20 per cent of all the blood and the oxygen output of the body, even a small blockage of a blood vessel can do a great deal of harm.

Both exercise and an effective diet can reduce the risks of blood vessel diseases. This is true even in such a serious problem as congestive heart failure, in which the weakened heart cannot pump sufficient blood, as exercise can improve the sufferer's endurance and heart strength. Studies at the Free University of Berlin have shown a 65 per cent increase in fitness after only three weeks of exercise.[3]

HARDENED ARTERIES AND HIGH BLOOD PRESSURE

Hardened arteries (atherosclerosis) and high blood pressure (hypertension) go hand-in-hand as the major contributors to both heart disease and stroke. Arteries become less efficient when their inner linings thicken and are roughened by deposits of fat, fibrin, cellular debris and calcium. The resulting reduction in the diameter of the blood vessels slows the blood flow, making it easier for clots to form and further restrict the blood flow of the arteries. Atherosclerosis is responsible for about 95 per cent of all heart attacks.

Fatty deposits on the artery walls (atherosclerosis) may begin as tumours which accumulate fat. These tumours may result from a genetic defect in the cell. The defect may then be stimulated into growth by outside influences such as high blood pressure (hypertension), cigarette smoking, free oxygen radicals, items in the diet or possibly viruses.

Hypertension is the primary indicator of heart attack, stroke and kidney disease. Many millions of people have it. More than half of them are not aware of their condition because there are usually no symptoms. Blacks are particularly prone to this condition, being afflicted three times more often than whites.

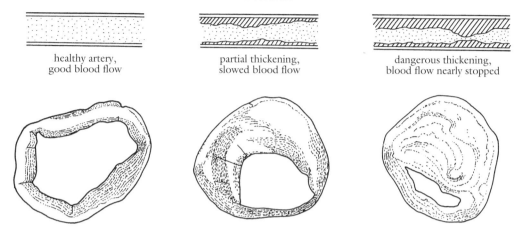

atherosclerosis

healthy artery,
good blood flow

partial thickening,
slowed blood flow

dangerous thickening,
blood flow nearly stopped

Fig 3. Cross-sectional views of *(from left)* a healthy artery, a partially thickened artery, and a badly diseased artery.

Hypertension is of concern because of the harm it can do to the heart, kidneys, brain and blood vessels if it remains uncontrolled for long periods of time. The heart is the organ most commonly damaged by high blood pressure. The increased force required during each beat makes the heart muscle thicken and become abnormally enlarged. It also speeds the hardening of the arteries of the heart.

High blood pressure occurs when the blood vessels in the body are constricted, either by nervous impulse or a build-up of plaque in the arteries. The heart is then required to beat more forcefully than normal. This forceful beat increases the pressure of the blood flowing from the heart.

Among the causes for hypertension are: a narrowing of the arteries, a tumour on the adrenal gland, kidney disease, obstructions in the arteries to the kidneys, and diabetes. These can usually be surgically or medically corrected. Approximately 90 per cent of all high blood pressure cannot be attributed to any one cause. Heredity, obesity, diet (particularly excess salt or inadequate potassium), smoking and anxiety may each play a part, as can alcohol consumption. Some drugs can also raise blood pressure, such as steroids, caffeine, drugs with stimulants (such as some cold remedies, nasal decongestants and appetite suppressants), and some depressants.

The effects of the disease include: kidney damage, artery wall damage, artery wall aneurysms (bulges) or haemorrhage, which is often a cause of strokes, and the development of atherosclerotic plaques in the arteries of the heart and brain.

Your blood pressure is easily checked. Sphygmomanometers (Greek for pulse pressure measurer) and stethoscopes can be bought inexpensively at any medical supply house. Some have the stethoscope built into the sphygmomanometer, making it very easy to take one's own blood pressure. Electronic sphygmomanometers are the simplest to use. Your blood pressure is measured by two

19

numbers. Every beat of your heart pushes a wave of blood through your blood vessels, which raises the pressure in the arteries. This is called systolic blood pressure and is represented by the first number. The blood pressure

Take your Blood Pressure

1. Wrap the cuff around your upper arm, just above the elbow.
2. Tighten the screw on the rubber bulb so that you can pump up the cuff.
3. Place the stethoscope on the inside of the elbow, just below the biceps muscle (this is where the artery passes).
4. While listening for a heartbeat with the stethoscope, pump up the cuff. When the gauge shows between 70 and 100mm of mercury, you should hear your pulse.
5. Continue pumping the cuff until you cannot hear the pulse, perhaps to 140 to 160mm of mercury. Then slowly let the air out of the cuff by twisting the valve on the air pump.
6. When you hear your heart beat through the stethoscope, note the number on the gauge. This is your systolic pressure (the pressure of your blood when the heart beats).
7. Continue to let the air out of the cuff. When you no longer hear your heart beat, note the number on the gauge. This is your diastolic pressure (the pressure while the heart is relaxing).

Blood pressure is recorded thus:

$$\frac{\text{systolic pressure}}{\text{diastolic pressure}}$$

Normal blood pressure is approximately:

$$\frac{120}{80}$$

The diastolic pressure is more important. It may be significant if it is continually higher.

Stages of Hypertension

Your **systolic pressure** (pressure at the time your heart is contracting) is the higher number. Your **diastolic pressure** (the continuous pressure at the time your heart is recovering from its contraction) is the lower number.

- Up to 130/up to 85 is in the normal range – but lower is better.
- 130–139/85–89 is high normal blood pressure
- 140–159/90–99 is considered mild hypertension (stage 1)
- 160–179/100–109 is moderate hypertension (stage 2)
- 180–209/110–119 is severe hypertension (stage 3)
- 210 and higher/120 and higher is very severe hypertension (stage 4)

If your systolic pressure and your diastolic pressures are in different categories, consider yourself in the higher (worse) category.

(Source: *Report of the Joint National Committee on Detection, Evaluation, and Treatment of High Blood Pressure*, Bethesda, MD: National Heart, Lung, and Blood Institute, National High Blood Pressure Program, 1993.)

between heartbeats, when the heart is recovering, is called the diastolic pressure and is the second and lower number.

The more desirable blood pressure is between 110/70 to 120/80. The numbers represent the number of millimetres of mercury which are being lifted in the sphygmomanometer by the pressure of the blood.

The figure 110/70 is ideal and is normal for many women, and many experts would like to have this measure considered to be normal for all. However, 120/80 is generally considered to be normal and is common for many men;

140/90 is borderline high. Generally, lower is better – unless it gets so low that you faint.

This may happen when it reaches 90/60 or below. Some research is now questioning the 'lower is better' concept because there is evidence that heart attack risk may elevate when the diastolic level is below 74.[4] Research to determine the validity of this theory and its possible causes is currently being conducted.

Blood pressure may vary greatly during any one day, so a high reading is not conclusive, but if it remains high, it may be dangerous – and a doctor should be consulted. Having a sphygmomanometer at home makes it easy to get an accurate picture of your blood pressure. One in six homes in the US already have them.

The danger of high blood pressure can be seen if we understand that a person whose systolic blood pressure is over 150 has twice the risk of heart attack and four times the risk of stroke as a person with a systolic pressure under 120. Insurance companies' studies show that a 35 year-old with a blood pressure of 145/95 will live 12 years less than someone with normal blood pressure.

THE CAUSES OF VASCULAR PROBLEMS

It seems that the same factors are related in the development of both atherosclerosis and hypertension. It is likely that either one may cause the other. Thus their possible causes will be discussed together.

Heredity

Heredity is often responsible for the tendency to high blood pressure and for being overweight. In studies comparing children of both natural and adoptive parents, the parents with abnormal body weight or blood pressure gave birth to children who manifested the same symptoms. Adopted children in the same household tended to have normal readings despite identical diets.

Inherited racial characteristics may also play a part. Among blacks, one in four has hypertension (only one in 500 has the much publicized sickle-cell anaemia). Among whites, one person in eight is hypertensive. Whether inherited or environmentally induced, our blood pressures seem to be determined, to a large degree, early in our lives.

Environment

Our environment is also a major cause of cardiovascular disease. Being overweight, eating certain types of foods, reactions to stress, cigarette smoking and inadequate exercise are all possible contributors to cardiovascular diseases.

Exercise

Exercise which requires that the heart works hard for a reasonably long period of time is a positive factor in keeping the circulatory system functioning efficiently. There are various theories as to why it works, but the results of effective exercise are well established. Exercise aids in reducing the effects of stress, lowers harmful blood fats while raising the protective blood fats, and may increase the number of open blood vessels in the heart. These combined effects not only lessen the possibility of a heart attack, they also increase one's chances of survival should a heart attack occur.

Moderate exercise can improve your heart's health significantly. Walking is the activity of choice for many heart patients. The recommended 'dosage' is 12 to 15 miles (19–24 km) per week, but start at whatever distance is comfortable for you, and gradually increase the distance over weeks and months. Such exercise can reduce your body weight and

21

blood pressure and can make your heart more efficient by slowing the pulse rate and increasing the amount of blood pumped during each heartbeat.[5]

A recent Dutch study which took twenty sedentary men and fourteen sedentary women, then trained them by having them walk and run three or four times a week for nine months, culminating in them running a half-marathon (13 miles/21km), found significant changes in their bodies which resulted from their training. The men lost an average of 5lb (2.3kg) and the women 2.5lb (1.1kg). The men had significant reductions in their total cholesterol, their low density lipoproteins (LDLs – the most dangerous of the cholesterols) and their triglycerides, all of which are greatly associated with heart attack risk.[6] The reduction in risk factors was much greater in the men than in the women, but this is partially accounted for by the female hormones which reduce the female risk until the menopause.

A British study of nearly 10,000 male civil servants with no history of heart disease was followed for nearly ten years. During that time, 474 experienced a heart attack. Of those who had reported that they exercised vigorously (cycling, running or fast walking at over 4mph (6.4km/h)), only half of the rate of heart problems occurred. Those who exercised less but still somewhat vigorously, had a two-thirds risk compared to the non-exercisers. The exercise had to be vigorous and aerobic.[7]

Smoking

Smoking has many negative effects which make the circulatory system less efficient. The smoker raises both blood pressure and blood fats. The carbon monoxide in the blood makes the blood less efficient. This makes the heart work much harder to circulate the required oxygen to the body. Smoking is directly responsible for between 100,000 and 200,000 heart attack deaths each year in the United States and even more in Europe. But 5 to 10 years after quitting, the risk is back to the level of those who have never smoked.[8] In one major study, people with problems who then stopped smoking enjoyed a 62 per cent reduction in deaths over the next 6 years compared to those who continued to smoke.[9]

Overweight

Excess body fat also increases the work of the heart. Every pound of fat (0.5kg) adds about 200 miles (322km) of capillaries which must be filled with blood so that the fat can be nourished. Being overweight increases the risk of high blood pressure, high blood cholesterol and diabetes.

Stress

Stress may be a factor in cardiovascular diseases. The classic study in this area was done by Doctors Meyer Friedman and Ray Rosenman. They brought great insight into the evaluation of stress when they coined the terms Type A and Type B personalities.[10] They cited several characteristics that show up in high-risk heart patients. They found that these high-risk people have a severe sense of time urgency – they want to get things done. They are constantly involved in multiple projects subject to deadlines. They have a desire for recognition and advancement and an excessive competitive drive. They neglect all aspects of life except work. They have a tendency to take on excessive responsibilities, feeling that, 'Only I can handle it'. Their speech patterns show explosiveness and a tendency to hasten the pace of their normal conversation.

Type A people are excessively ambitious, expressing overwhelming aggression and impatience, and are slaves to the clock. They are the competitive types who may even compete with themselves – such as pushing themselves to improve their time while running, jogging or swimming. They drive themselves excessively, don't take holidays, walk fast, talk fast and are compulsive. They are concerned with making money, and they compete in just about everything they do.

The Type B personalities may be just as serious about where they are going, but they are easy-going, seldom impatient, and they take time out for leisure. They don't feel driven by the clock to get things done. They are not preoccupied with social achievement and are less competitive. This personality type may be easily sidetracked because they are not as intense in their drive to accomplish. Studies have shown that the Type A personality is two to three times as likely to have a heart attack as the Type B personality.

More recently, theorists have looked at the Type A people and have concluded that it may not be their ambitious natures as much as their competitiveness which increases their heart attack risk. The Type As without hostility seemed to live as long as Type Bs, whereas the Type As were more prone to heart attacks.

The physiological effects of negative stress situations are reflected in higher blood pressure and the secretion of more adrenaline. Both of these are known risk factors for heart problems. Negative stress has also been shown to increase the stickiness of the blood platelets and make them more likely to clot.[11] In the Framingham study, anxiety levels in middle-aged men, but not women, were predictive of hypertension.[12] In another study, high-stress men 'outdied' their low-stress counterparts by a three to one ratio over a five-year period.

On the other hand, studies at the Institute of Gerontology in Kiev indicate that the easy life may shorten life spans. Studies done there with animals at the molecular level, the cell level and the systemic level revealed that animals subjected to certain stresses lived longer than those experiencing ideal conditions. These Russian researchers believe that the key to long life may be in the hypothalamus. They found that cell nuclei of this gland age at different rates for different people.

Dr Hans Selye, director of the Institute of Experimental Medicine and Surgery at the University of Montreal, and perhaps the world's leading authority on stress, said that, 'It is not the stress that is the problem, but how one reacts to stress. The trick is not to avoid stress, but to enjoy and master it.'

Stress is often related to not being in control of one's situation. Those in the lower social classes are also at the bottom of their job classifications. Those in the bottom 10 per cent of job classifications have four to five times the number of heart attacks compared to those at the top 10 per cent of the job ladder.[13]

Finally, when faced with stressful situations, learn to respond with thought-out solutions and avoid anger and hostility rather than resort to knee-jerk reactions. Recognize that overreacting to things you cannot control can be harmful to your heart's health.

Diet

This is an area which has been studied at great depth. In addition to the positive effects of low fat diets and diets low in sodium and high in potassium, the addition of antioxidants is being increasingly recognized as an important step in reducing both heart disease and many cancers. Vitamins C and E and beta carotene, which is converted into vitamin A, as well as the mineral selenium, all have antioxidant properties which are thought to reduce the damage in the artery walls that precedes the development of the atherosclerotic plaques in the arteries.

People who live in parts of the world which are rich in selenium, a trace mineral found in

23

soil, plants and water, are much less likely to die of heart attacks, strokes, aneurysms and other problems related to high blood pressure. This mineral is sometimes included among the antioxidants. However, it has been found to be toxic in higher doses. European soil is low in selenium so it should be supplemented.[14]

Moderate alcohol consumption, particularly some red wines, also seems to be a preventative for heart disease. It raises the HDL lipids which carry cholesterol away from the tissues and back to the liver. Of course, there are some negatives associated with alcohol, including the increased calorie intake and the possible toxic effects on other organs.[15]

Fats in the Blood

These are considered to be the prime contributors to hardened arteries. The most studied blood fats are the lipoproteins, cholesterols and triglycerides.

The major types of lipoproteins are:

- heavy density lipoproteins (HDL), which transport cholesterol from the body's tissues to the liver where it can be eliminated;
- low density lipoproteins (LDL), which take cholesterol from the liver to the tissues; these contain few triglycerides. 60 to 80 per cent of the body's cholesterol is carried by the LDL; and
- very low density lipoproteins (VLDL), which contain primarily triglycerides with a little cholesterol. They carry triglycerides to the tissues and fat of the body, where they can be used for energy.

Cholesterol is a waxy substance used in many of the body's chemical processes. It is required by everyone in certain amounts, but when there is too much cholesterol being carried by the LDLs some may be deposited in the artery walls. This is the build-up which we call atherosclerosis (artery 'fat scarring' or hardened arteries).

Cholesterols are derived primarily from saturated fats that are eaten in the diet and from cholesterol which is ingested. About 70 to 80 per cent of cholesterol is made in the body, primarily by the liver, from saturated fats that are eaten; the remaining 20 to 30 per cent of the blood's cholesterol is eaten in the form of cholesterol in animal products.

The amount of cholesterol in your blood is measured as millimoles per litre (mmol/l) in Europe and as milligrams per decilitre (mg/dl) in the United States.

It is highly recommended that all people have a total blood evaluation when they are young. This can give a 'base line' level against which future examinations can be measured. It can also reveal any dangerously high levels of one of the blood fats. The recommended

---

Measurement of Cholesterol

Americans use a cholesterol measurement that is different from most other countries. The doctors in the United States use milligrams per decilitre (mg/dl). Most other countries use millimoles per litre (mmol/l). A millimole is a thousandth of a mole.

To convert US values (mg/dl) to other values (mmol/l) divide the US value by 38.5.

To convert the other values to US values multiply the other value by 38.5.

Thus:

- desirable level would be under 200 (mg/dl) or 5.2 (mmol/l).
- borderline high would be 200 to 239 (mg/dl) or 5.2 to 6.19 (mmol/l).
- high would be over 240 (mg/dl) or 6.2 (mmol/l).

total blood cholesterol level is below 5.19mmol/l (200mg/dl) with 3.9mmol/l (150mg/dl) being considered to be ideal. Lower is better. In the Framingham study in Massachusetts, the classic study in the field of heart disease, there have been 5,209 adults involved in the programme since 1948. In correlating all the factors that relate to heart disease, it was found that the cholesterol levels of the blood are a primary determinant in predicting heart attack risk.

People with blood cholesterol levels over 6.63mmol/l (255mg/dl) of blood have five times the heart attack risk as those with the level of 5.72 Europe (220 USA). Men, whose cholesterol level was 5.98 Europe (230 USA), suffered three times as many heart attacks as men with cholesterol levels under 5.46 Europe (210 USA). It is generally considered that for every 0.026 mmol/l (1 point mg/cu. cm3 in US) you drop in your cholesterol level that you reduce your chances of dying by 2 per cent.

The saturated fats, from which cholesterol is made, are found primarily in the animal fats contained in beef, lamb, pork, ham, whole milk, cream, butter and whole milk cheeses (the hard cheeses). But they are also found in vegetable fats which are solid or which have been hydrogenated (trans-fatty acids) such as shortenings, coconut oil, cocoa butter and palm oil (which is used in commercially prepared biscuits and pie fillings). They are also found in non-dairy milk and cream substitutes and in chocolate.

While people commonly talk about 'good' and 'bad' cholesterol, it is really the carrier of the cholesterol which is good or bad depending on whether they are taking the cholesterol to the liver or away from the liver and into the tissues – including the arteries.

The *HDLs* (the 'good' lipoproteins) are associated with lower cardiovascular risk because they are able to get rid of the cholesterols which, if allowed to stay in the blood, can develop plaques in the arteries of the heart, neck and brain. These then increase the risk of heart attack and stroke. Women tend to have more HDL than men due to the oestrogen they produce. Oestrogen replacement after menopause can continue this protection, otherwise women's heart attack risk rates will rise as they grow older.

While polyunsaturated oils had previously been advocated in the bid to reduce blood cholesterol, we now know that they also lower the HDL. For this reason, the monounsaturated fats, such as those found in olive oil and rapeseed oil, are more often recommended as a source of fat.[16] Stopping smoking, maintaining a proper weight and exercising effectively are all ways in which HDLs may be raised.

The HDL levels should be higher than 0.91 Europe (35mg/dl USA) for men and over 1.69 Europe (65mg/dl USA) for women. Higher is better. A level below 0.91 (35) is a very negative risk factor. Another important measure is the ratio of total cholesterol to HDL. It is derived by dividing the HDL level into the total cholesterol level. It should be less than three for women and less than four for men.

The *LDLs* (the 'bad' lipoproteins) carry cholesterol to the tissues. Some of this may be implanted in the arteries, hardening and narrowing them. This process seems to need oxygenation to occur. It is the free oxygen radicals which change the fat in the LDL. Once changed, it can then be deposited into the artery walls. Both HDL and the antioxidant vitamins (A, C, and E) reduce the rate of this oxygenation.[17] Vitamin E supplementation of 100 I.U. per day reduced women's risk of heart attack by 33 per cent and men's by 25 per cent.[18] Dr Ken Cooper, of aerobics fame, suggests 400 I.U. per day of vitamin E. The previously mentioned polyunsaturated fats increase the likelihood of oxygenation. The top normal level for LDL is 3.64mmol/l (140mg/dl), and it is desirable to have it under 338 (130). Lower is better. *See* Chapter 9 for more on free oxygen radicals and antioxidants.

A Swedish study, sponsored by Volvo, showed that generally women have less LDL than men but, as they move up the occupational scale, their levels approach that of men. However, while the more competitive Type A men had a much higher level than Type B men, the Type A and B women had similar levels in each job category. The HDL levels for women remained higher than men at every level.[19]

Triglycerides are the most common type of blood fat. While they are found in some foods, such as luncheon meats and shellfish, they are generally constructed in the liver from carbohydrates, such as sugars, in the diet. Although we hear much more about cholesterol in the blood, some experts think that the triglycerides may be even more harmful than the cholesterols.[20]

Blood tests for triglycerides and blood cholesterol should be part of everyone's physical examination from the age of three. The normal level for triglycerides is 1.3 to 3.9 Europe (50–150 USA), but the lower the better. Endurance (aerobic) exercise has been found to reduce triglycerides (because they are used for energy during the exercise). It also increases the amount of HDL.

Heredity can also play a part in the body's ability to produce too much cholesterol or triglycerides. When heredity is the problem, either drug therapy or surgery may be required to eliminate the problem. Even when diet and a lack of exercise are the primary problems, drug therapy can often be used to reduce the blood levels of these fats.

It is the combination of risk factors that increases one's chances of developing a cardiovascular disease, especially coronary artery disease. To the degree that coronary artery disease is increased, the risk of heart attack is also increased.

Two members of the Harvard University School of Public Health have reported a study of the health records of 50,000 former students at Harvard and at the University of Pennsylvania in respect to fatal heart attacks and heart attack risks. The study revealed that 1,146 of the former students died between the ages of 30 and 69 years from fatal heart attacks. When these students were compared with classmates who had not suffered heart attacks, the scientists found six clues or relationships that increased the risk of death from heart attack. These relationships were as follows:

1. Cigarette smoking. Smoking in college was found to be associated with a 50 per cent increased risk of a coronary death.
2. Non-participation in sports. The college student who engaged in no sports while in college was found to have a 50 per cent increase in his risk of a fatal heart attack.
3. An elevated blood pressure. A systolic blood pressure in excess of 130mm Hg while in college was found to be associated with a 40 per cent increase in the risk of death from heart attack.
4. Heavier than average body weight. Excessive body weight for height was found to increase the risk of an eventual fatal heart attack by 30 per cent.
5. A height of less than 5ft 6in (168cm). Short stature was found by investigators to be associated with an increase of 30 per cent in the risk of death from heart disease.
6. Early death of a parent. The early death of a parent (based on deaths from all causes) was associated with a 30 per cent greater chance of dying from a heart attack.

From this, we might infer that the person who smokes cigarettes, is inactive physically, has a slightly elevated blood pressure, is short and overweight, and who has the heredity for a

American Heart Association's Heart Attack Risk Test for Those Who Know Their Cholesterol and Blood Pressure Levels

Age for Men		*Age for Women*	
Less than 35	0 points	Less than 42	0 points
35 to 39	1 point	42 to 44	1 point
40 to 48	2 points	45 to 54	2 points
49 to 53	3 points	55 to 73	3 points
54 or older	4 points	74 or older	4 points

Family History
Someone in your family had heart disease or a heart attack before age 60 2 points _____

Inactive Lifestyle
Rarely exercise   1 point _____

Weight
More than 20lb (9kg) over ideal weight   1 point _____

Smoking
I am a smoker   1 point _____

Diabetic
Male diabetic   1 point _____
Female diabetic   2 points _____

Total cholesterol level
Less than 240mg/dl (6.23 mmol/l)   0 points _____
240 to 315mg/dl (6.23 to 8.18 mmol/l)   1 point _____
above 315mg/dl (8.18 mmol/l   2 points _____

HDL level (good cholesterol)
Over 60mg/dl (1.56 mmol/l)   subtract 1 point _____
39 to 59mg/dl (1 to 1.53 mmol/l)   0 points _____
30-38mg/dl (0.78 to 1 mmol/l)   1point _____
Under 30mg/dl (0.78 mmol/l)   2 points _____

Blood Pressure
If you take blood pressure medicine   1 point _____
If you do not take blood pressure medicine
and your systolic (the higher) number is: Less than 140   0 points _____
                                               140 to 170   1 point _____
                                               Over 170   2 points _____

TOTAL POINTS _____
(4 points and over indicates a
higher than normal risk for a
first heart attack.)

shorter life, is the person of today who is most likely to suffer a fatal heart attack in the future.

Other risk factors which have been shown to be related to heart attack and to death from the attack are: depression, anger and living alone. These factors also multiplied the effects of other risk factors. For example, for smokers who were also depressed, the amount of artery hardening was nearly three and a half times greater than in non-depressed smokers. And LDL levels were twice as high for depressives as for non-depressed people.[21]

You can aid in preventing or slowing the progress of cardiovascular disease. To slow the hardening of the arteries and to minimize the chances of developing heart disease and strokes, it is wise to keep your blood pressure low and your blood fats in the proper proportions.

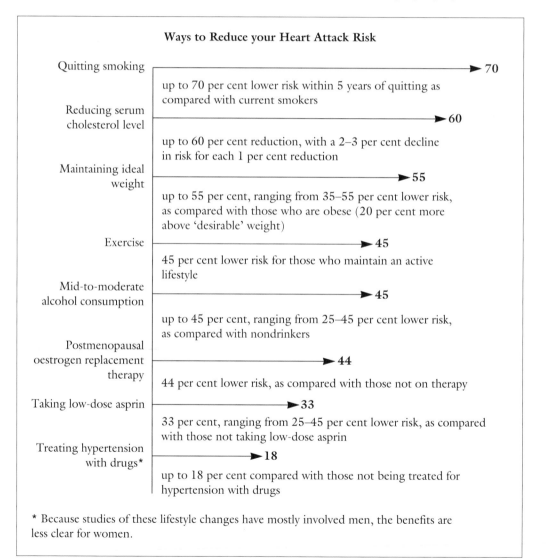

Ways to Reduce your Heart Attack Risk

Quitting smoking — 70
up to 70 per cent lower risk within 5 years of quitting as compared with current smokers

Reducing serum cholesterol level — 60
up to 60 per cent reduction, with a 2–3 per cent decline in risk for each 1 per cent reduction

Maintaining ideal weight — 55
up to 55 per cent, ranging from 35–55 per cent lower risk, as compared with those who are obese (20 per cent more above 'desirable' weight)

Exercise — 45
45 per cent lower risk for those who maintain an active lifestyle

Mid-to-moderate alcohol consumption — 45
up to 45 per cent, ranging from 25–45 per cent lower risk, as compared with nondrinkers

Postmenopausal oestrogen replacement therapy — 44
44 per cent lower risk, as compared with those not on therapy

Taking low-dose asprin — 33
33 per cent, ranging from 25–45 per cent lower risk, as compared with those not taking low-dose asprin

Treating hypertension with drugs* — 18
up to 18 per cent compared with those not being treated for hypertension with drugs

* Because studies of these lifestyle changes have mostly involved men, the benefits are less clear for women.

Your risk of having a heart attack is determined by many factors. The game 'Risko', developed by the Michigan Heart Association, may be of value to you in evaluating some of these risk factors.

This game is not a complete measurement of risk factors, since it is very difficult to measure things such as diabetes, the stress factor under which you live, the vital capacity of your lungs, the actual condition of your heart, and whether or not you have gout. These things can only be done by a doctor, but the game can give you some idea as to your general risk of suffering a heart attack.

The game is played by making squares which – from left to right (*see* overleaf) – represent an increase in your *risk factors*. These are medical conditions and habits associated with an increased danger of heart attack. Not all risk factors are measurable enough to be included in this game.

RULES

Study each *risk factor* and its row. Find the box applicable to you and circle the large number in it. For example, if you are 37, circle the number in the box labelled 31–40.

After checking all the rows, add the circled numbers. This total – your score – is an estimate of your risk.

If you score:
6 to 11 – Risk well below average   25 to 31 – Risk moderate
12 to 17 – Risk below average   32 to 40 – Risk at a dangerous level
18 to 24 – Risk generally average   41 to 62 – Danger urgent. See your doctor now

Heredity:
Count parents, grandparents, brothers and sisters who have had a heart attack and/or stroke.

Tobacco Smoking:
If you inhale deeply and smoke all of a cigarette, add one to your classification. Do *not* subtract because you think you do not inhale or smoke only half an inch of a cigarette.

Exercise:
Lower your score one point if you exercise regularly.

Cholesterol or Saturated Fat Intake Level:
A cholesterol blood level test is best. If you can not get one from your doctor, then estimate honestly the percentage of solid fats you eat. These are usually of animal origin – lard, cream, butter and beef and lamb fat. If you eat a high proportion of this, your cholesterol level will probably be high. Keep saturated fat intake to under 10 per cent of diet.

Blood Pressure:
If you have no recent reading but have passed an insurance or industrial examination the chances are that you are 140 or less.

Sex:
This line takes into account the fact that men have from six to ten times more heart attacks than women of child-bearing age.

(continued overleaf)

Self-Test (continued)

	10 to 20 (1)	21 to 30 (2)	31 to 40 (3)	41 to 50 (4)	51 to 60 (6)	61 to 70 and over (8)
Age						
Heredity	No known history of heart disease (1)	1 relative over 60 with cardiovascular disease (2)	2 relatives over 60 with cardiovascular disease (3)	1 relative under 60 with cardiovascular disease (4)	2 relatives under 60 with cardiovascular disease (6)	3 relatives under 60 with cardiovascular disease (7)
Weight	More than 5lb (2.3kg) below standard weight (0)	−5 to +5lb (−2.3 to +2.3kg) standard weight (1)	6–20lb (2.7–9kg) overweight (2)	21–35lb (9.5–16kg) overweight (3)	36–50lb (16.3–22.6kg) overweight (5)	51–65lb (23–29.5kg) overweight (7)
Tobacco smoking	Non-user (0)	Cigar and/or pipe (1)	10 cigarettes or less a day (2)	20 cigarettes a day (4)	30 cigarettes a day (6)	40 cigarettes a day or more (10)
Exercise	Intensive occupational and recreational exertion (1)	Moderate occupational and recreational exertion (2)	Sedentary work and intense recreational exertion (3)	Sedentary occupational and moderate recreational exertion (5)	Sedentary work and light recreational exertion (6)	Complete lack of exercise (8)
Cholesterol or fat % in diet	Cholesterol below 180mg.%. Diet contains no animal or solid fats (1)	Cholesterol 181–205mg.%. Diet contains 10% animal or solid fats (2)	Cholesterol 206–230mg.%. Diet contains 20% animal or solid fats (3)	Cholesterol 231–255mg.%. Diet contains 30% animal or solid fats (4)	Cholesterol 256–280mg.%. Diet contains 40% animal or solid fats (5)	Cholesterol 281–300mg.%. Diet contains 50% animal or solid fats (7)
Blood pressure	100 upper reading (1)	120 upper reading (2)	140 upper reading (3)	160 upper reading (4)	180 upper reading (6)	200 or over upper reading (8)
Sex	Female under 40 (1)	Female 40–50 (2)	Female over 50 (3)	Male (5)	Stocky male (6)	Bald, stocky male (7)

Total points _____

(Michigan Heart Foundation)

In order to begin to do this, it is suggested that you have a physical examination. This will assist in spotting high blood pressure and high cholesterol or high triglyceride levels in the blood. It will also find heart irregularities through the use of the stethoscope and the electrocardiogram. For every 1 per cent you reduce your blood pressure or your cholesterol, you reduce your heart attack risk by 2 to 3 per cent.

Your eating habits can assist in controlling general body weight, and the lower your body weight, the less your chances are of developing heart disease. You can lower your fat intake. Our average diet consists of about 35 to 45 per cent fat. It is suggested that the fat intake should be between 10 and 20 per cent of the total calories. Cholesterol intake should be below 300 milligrams per day.

Salt intake should also be reduced. There seems to be a direct relationship between the amount of salt in the diet and the incidence of high blood pressure. In the northern islands of Japan, the diet is twice as high in salt as in southern Japan. The frequency of high blood pressure is also twice as high. In Western societies we consume about ten times as much sodium as is necessary. It would be a good idea to take the salt shaker off the table and to avoid highly salted, processed foods.

Vitamin supplementation, while once frowned upon, is now often recommended. Higher levels of the antioxidants, vitamins C, E and beta carotene and a little selenium, are common recommendations.[22]

Taking half an aspirin daily is also recommended by those who suffer no ill effects from the aspirin. The aspirin reduces the blood's ability to clot, thereby the risk of a thrombus or embolism forming. Omega 3 oil from some fish is also recommended because it reduces the blood's ability to clot and seems to reduce the level of LDLs.

One or two glasses of alcohol per day may be beneficial in reducing the risk of heart attack, but it must be weighed against the possible detrimental effects of increased calories and the possible increase of hypertension. For people who have had heart problems, the drinking of alcohol may be hazardous. Patients with heart disease may be extraordinarily susceptible to myocardial depression (a weakening of the heart muscle action) which is a result of alcohol. Patients with severe cardiac damage and chronic congestive heart failure should probably not drink at all.

Exercise improves the cardiovascular efficiency by increasing the amount of oxygen-carrying red cells in each unit of blood. It often lowers blood cholesterol and may widen the blood vessels of the heart. It also seems to decrease the effects of stress.

Stopping smoking is extremely important in the prevention of heart disease. When you stop smoking, your blood pressure will generally lower, the amount of oxygen in each unit of blood will be increased, the artery hardening process will slow down, and the amount of cholesterol in the blood will be reduced.

Taking quiet times during the day, which can reduce one's stress, may also be beneficial. Dr Herbert Benson, Associate Professor of Medicine at Harvard University, studied transcendental meditation. He found that prayer or meditation may promote the peace of mind which can reduce stress.

CHAPTER 4
Cancer

Cancer causes 16 per cent of all deaths. Half of these deaths will occur before the people reach 65 years ago. Cancer is more than one disease. In fact, it is probably a hundred different diseases. A simple definition of cancer is that it amounts to the uncontrolled growth of abnormal cells. For some reason not yet understood, these cells break away from the normal restraining influences of the body's systems. This uncontrolled growth can impinge on vital organs and block blood vessels by growing to such a mass that tumours develop. A recent theory hinges on the idea that it is not so much that the cells multiply, but that they do not die. A gene has been identified which is part of the immune system and which seems to keep some immune cells alive so that they can 'remember' past infections. It is hypothesized that if too many cells are instructed not to die, cancer may be a result.

Tumours can be benign (harmless) or malignant (harmful and spreading). A wart or a cyst would be an example of a benign tumour. Malignant, uncontrolled cancers can either be carcinomas, sarcomas, lymphomas or leukaemias:

- The carcinomas originate in the linings of the tissues, the epithelial cells such as the skin, the mucus membranes and the intestinal linings.
- The sarcomas develop in the muscle, bone, cartilage and fibrous tissues. These are less common.
- Lymphomas begin in a lymph node.
- Leukaemias are problems in the blood producing bone marrows and the resultant increase in certain white blood cells which spread through the body.

Once a cancer begins, the cells can travel from one place to another by penetrating the walls, the veins of lymph channels. They can then travel with the blood or the lymph to areas that were far distant from their point of origin. This is called metastasis. Many cancers have travelled to distant points of the body before the original cancer is diagnosed. When regional involvement develops there is much less chance of curing the cancer, and if the regional involvement is extensive, death is almost inevitable but not always quick.

Heredity is generally not a cause of cancer, although there is a form of eye cancer which is apparently inherited. However, heredity may predispose a person to cancer. For example, very fair skin would predispose a person to skin cancer from the sun's rays. Cancer does tend to run in families. Several genes have been found which are linked to either the development of cancer cells or the inability of the body to recognize the cells so that they can be destroyed.

Environmental causes are responsible for 60 to 90 per cent of all cancers. Such factors as air pollution, smoking, water pollution, chemicals, foods, radiation, dust, asbestos fibres and charcoal can be carcinogenic.

The environmental aspects of cancer can be illustrated by the increased breast cancer and leukaemia rates of the people who lived in Hiroshima and Nagasaki after the atom bombs were dropped. The leukaemia rate (blood cancer) of survivors of Hiroshima and Nagasaki was five times as high as for those people in the Japanese population as a whole. The effect of radiation is shown in the leukaemia rates for X-ray workers. It is also seen in the skin cancer rates for people exposed to the sun, such as farmers and sailors.

Chemical agents such as alcohol, cigarette smoke and soot may have caused cancers of the digestive system, the lungs and the scrotum. Scrotal cancer is a characteristic found among chimney sweeps in England where they were exposed to the soot of the chimneys.

Only 6,000 of the 2,000,000 known chemicals have been tested for cancer-causing potential. Of these, 50 per cent have already been found to be cancer producing. For example, it is known that there is a link between lung cancer and the handling of asbestos or to exposure to fumes in coking plants. The connection between bladder cancer and exposure to benzene in the rubber and dye industries has also been established.

In 1975, three US scientists shared the Nobel Prize for Physiology and Medicine for their research into possible links between viruses and cancer. However, one of them, Dr Howard Temin of the University of Wisconsin, who did studies linking a type of virus to cancer in chickens, said that he believes that the majority of human cancers are not primarily caused by infectious viruses, but by radiation and chemicals.

Certain cancers are caused when normal cells are turned into cancer cells. Very often, these cancers need certain amino acids (the building blocks of proteins) in order to grow.

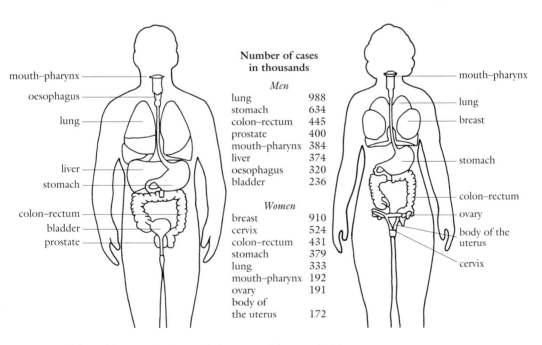

Fig 4. World Health Organization statistics on world cancer incidence.

Number of cases in thousands

Men

lung	988
stomach	634
colon–rectum	445
prostate	400
mouth–pharynx	384
liver	374
oesophagus	320
bladder	236

Women

breast	910
cervix	524
colon–rectum	431
stomach	379
lung	333
mouth–pharynx	192
ovary	191
body of the uterus	172

When these amino acids, especially phenylalanine and tryptophan, were eliminated from the diet, these certain cancers regressed. However, the elimination of those essential amino acids changed the people's sleep patterns. They dreamed less. They also lost weight because these essential amino acids are needed to build most tissues.

Cancers of the mouth, larynx, oesophagus and liver are definitely related to heavy alcohol consumption. A person who drinks more than three ounces of whisky, half a bottle of wine or four glasses of beer a day runs two and a half times the risk of developing mouth and throat cancer. Those who drink and smoke have fifteen times the risk of developing cancer of the mouth and throat compared to those who do neither.

SKIN CANCER

Skin cancer attacks one in one hundred people but its rate has nearly tripled in the last 20 years. There are about 7,000 deaths each year and 32,000 new cases diagnosed. But if diagnosed early, it can be controlled. Usually the lighter one's skin, the greater the danger. Blondes and redheads are more susceptible to skin cancer than brunettes, and blacks, Asians and Hispanics have only about 5 to 10 per cent of the risk of the lighter skinned people from northern Europe. Australians, who are exposed to 300 sunny days a year, have a very high rate of skin cancers – two out of three Australians will develop some form of the disease.

The worst skin damage occurs to those under 18. Severe sunburns early in life are correlated to serious cancers later in life, so it is particularly important to protect those who are younger. Young people may have to decide whether they want to look healthier when they are young or when they are older. So you might warn your grandchildren.

While most skin cancers are benign and easily removed, the deadly type, called melanoma, must be taken very seriously. If it is localized on the skin, the 5-year survival rate is 90 per cent but that survival rate drops to 55 per cent if the cancer has spread to nearby organs and to 14 per cent if it has spread to more distant organs.

The outer layer of skin, the epidermis, is made up of several types of cells which can be affected by the ultraviolet rays of the sun. Basal cell carcinoma is the most common type of skin cancer affecting 500,000 people each year. It sometimes metastasizes. Another type of skin cancer is squamous cell carcinoma. There are 100,000 cases of this type of cancer each year. It is caused not only by the sun's rays but also by hydrocarbons found in some oils, tars and asphalts.

There are several types of serious skin cancers (melanomas). Some appear as darker spots on the skin but the more serious are quite dark, such as moles, and are likely to have a rougher texture:

- Caucasians, particularly women, are likely to develop a melanoma which starts from a normal mole but which becomes irregular in both shape and size. This type accounts for 70 per cent of all cases.
- A second type is more common among Asians and Africans. The lesions are brown-black, blue-black or dark brown and are likely to occur on the hands, feet or mucous membranes.
- Another type is most common among women over 50 who have spent years in the sun.
- The lesions may appear to be blood blisters but their colours can range from nearly white to blue-black.

A monthly self-examination, preferably done with a friend, is the best way to spot an early cancer. Starting from the scalp, check for dark spots under the hair, on the face and neck, in the mouth, behind the ears, on the genitals, as well as on other parts of the body. A common place for such cancers to start in women is on the lower legs, so give them special attention.

The combination of a reduced ozone layer and more recreational hours spent in the sun is responsible for most skin cancers. This makes it more important than ever to wear sun protection with a sun protective factor (SPF) of at least fifteen. Make certain that it can block both the ultraviolet-A (UV-A) and the ultraviolet-B rays. It is wisest not to go into the sun when it is at its highest points (from 10a.m. to 3p.m.) and to avoid sun-tanning parlours. The UV-A rays of sun lamps and the sun can cause cancers just as the more dangerous UV-B radiation from the sun can. If your exercise or recreation programme takes you outdoors – such as jogging, rowing or lying on the beach – you should take the necessary precautions.

CANCER OF THE PROSTATE GLAND

Cancer of the prostate gland kills 38,000 of the more than 200,000 men who are diagnosed annually with the disease. It is the most common cancer among men. In men under 50, their chances of developing such a cancer are 5 per cent. In men over 50, it is 15 to 30 per cent, and by the time they are 70 years old, their chances are 50 per cent. Blacks also have a higher than normal risk of prostate cancer.

Smoking, alcohol use and particularly the fats in red meat are associated with increased risk. Such fats nearly tripled the amount of cancer which would be considered normal.

Men over 50 should have an annual prostate check. In this check a physician puts a gloved finger into the rectum and feels the prostate for unusual lumps. A blood test for prostate specific antigen (PSA) should also be done.

OVARIAN CANCER

Ovarian cancer is another cancer with strong hereditary links. It kills about 18,000 women annually. With no affected relatives the risk is one in seventy. With one close relative affected the risk is increased to one in twenty.

UTERINE CANCER

Uterine cancers kill about 14,000 women each year. The uterine cancers include cancer of the cervix, the uterus and the endometrial cancer which affects the body of the uterus. The Pap smear, named after its developer Dr George Papanicolaou, is a painless sampling of the cells of the cervix of the uterus. If cancer cells are present, the test detects them.

Cancer cells are measurable long before cancer becomes obvious and impossible to treat. The Pap smear has been responsible for a 65 per cent decline in uterine cancer. It is 95 per cent effective in determining cervical cancer but only 60 per cent effective in determining the endometrial cancer. This endometrial cancer is more likely to occur in older women, and its rate has been increasing rapidly in recent years. There is some evidence to indicate that the group in which it is increasing the most rapidly, white women over 50, may be those who are taking oestrogen to reduce the symptoms of the menopause. It is possible therefore that there is a relationship between endometrial cancer and oestrogen.

Women who have had irregular bleeding, spotting or other vaginal discharges are three times as likely to have a uterine cancer as women with no such problems. This is particularly true in women over 35 years old.

Many women have a benign type of tumour in the uterus called a fibroid. These growths usually shrink and disappear naturally after the menopause and do not often require surgical removal. For women over 35, a hysterectomy may be the best way of removing fibroids. Other tumours or cysts can occur on the ovaries. They are usually not malignant.

There is strong evidence that the herpes virus, similar to that which causes cold sores, causes both cervical cancer in women and prostate cancer in men. There is also evidence that it can be transferred sexually. One study showed that 15 per cent of men had herpes in their genito-urinary tracts. Herpes transfer can be minimized if the male wears a condom.

There has been found to be an 11 per cent incidence of cancer of the breasts and uteri in wives of men who have had prostatic cancer. For wives of men without prostatic cancer, the rate is only one per cent. This indicates that wives of men with prostate cancer should have breast and pelvic check-ups every six months.

Other correlations with cervical cancers found that the younger women are when they first experienced sexual intercourse, the greater their chances of developing cervical cancer. Among nuns, where you would expect no sexual experience, cervical cancer is virtually unknown. However, widowed women have 50 per cent more cervical cancer than married women, causing us to wonder. Divorced women, however, experience 72 per cent more cases of cervical cancer than married women. Jewish women only have one-ninth the chance of non-Jewish women of developing cervical cancer, possibly because Jewish males are circumcised, although there may be other reasons.

BREAST CANCER

Breast cancer will account for several hundred thousand new cases of cancer this year and hundreds of thousands of deaths in the Western world. If found and treated early, the five-year survival rate is 84 per cent. If it is found late, the survival rate is 56 per cent.

Genes which are linked to both ovarian and breast cancer have been discovered. BRCA 1 is located on the 17th chromosome and BRCA 2 is located on the 13th chromosome. These genes may be considered to be responsible for as many as 10 per cent of breast cancers.[1] Yet as many as 19 per cent of breast cancers may have a family history.[2] This study took into consideration not only mothers and sisters but more distant female relatives. Another study, while finding that a woman's risk was doubled if her mother was diagnosed with breast cancer before age 40, concluded that only 2.5 per cent of cases involved a family history of breast cancer. This study did not look at the more distant relatives.[3] Another genetic risk is race. Black women have a higher risk than whites until age 40, then their risk begins to drop.

Women who have not breast-fed their babies have two-thirds more risk of developing breast-cancer than those who have breast fed for at least 36 months. This indicates environmental causes. Alcohol consumption is another environmental risk, possibly because it increases oestrogen,[4] as is obesity after menopause. However, 70 per cent of women who develop this cancer have no known risk factors.

While the lifetime risk for developing a breast cancer is one in eight, the risk varies greatly with age. For those under 39 it is one in 217. From 40 to 59 it is 1 in twenty-six, and for women between 60 to 79 it is one in fifteen.[5]

Since two forms of oestrogen (oestradiol and progesterone) seem to be the culprits, any action which increases their production is a negative and any which reduces it is a positive. So early menstruation is a negative factor since the ovaries start producing these hormones early in life. Having a child and breast-feeding it reduces the levels of these hormones, as does aerobic exercise such as walking or running.

Breast cancers will not hurt, but they can often be detected. A simple breast check for

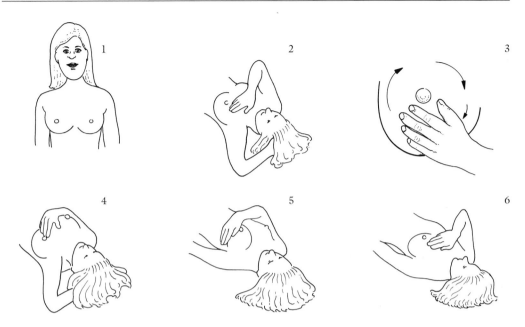

The best time to examine one's breasts is just after menstruation, when any swelling has subsided. Examining the breasts while bathing or showering, when the skin is wet and smooth, is also recommended.

Stand in front of a mirror and compare both breasts, looking for puckering or dimpling, any sores, pore enlargement, or orange-peel effects on the skin, and any obvious flattening or thickening. Squeeze the nipple to check for discharge, bloody or clear.

No two breasts look exactly alike, but marked differences, and any changes, should be noted. Leaning forward, placing the hands on the hips and flexing the chest muscles, and raising the hands over the head will accentuate any abnormalities. Then lie flat on your back with a cushion under the side to be examined, raising that arm overhead. Place the other hand gently but firmly over the breast and rotate the hand in a clockwise fashion. Do this at least three times, moving in towards the nipple, to make sure you have covered every part of the breast. Pay particular attention to the area adjacent to the armpit and to the armpit itself. Be particularly alert for any hard lumps – which may or may not appear to be movable. They will feel like a dried pea in a bowl of tapioca.

Repeat this procedure on the other breast. Report any abnormality to your doctor immediately.

Fig 5. Breast self-examination.

cancer can be done while lying down on the back with one hand behind the head. Curl the fingers of the other hand so that they conform to the shape of the breast. Run your fingers around the breast starting at approximately the '10 o'clock' position. Move the hand slowly around the breast in small and large circles and see if you find any nodules. Some nodules are normal glands; others could be pre-cancerous. You are looking for a dominant lump about the size of a small shirt button or larger.

After you have examined the breasts in the reclining position, examine them in the sitting position. Look for an enlargement of the skin pores or an orange-peel effect on the skin. Feel them for bulging or flattening in one breast which does not appear in the other. Look for a dimpling or puckering in the skin, a sore, a reddening or a crusty skin. See if there is a change in the appearance of the nipple, especially if it is pulled inwards. Squeeze the nipple gently to see if a discharge appears.

These breast cancer checks should be done throughout your lifetime since the chances of breast cancer increase with age.

As the initial cancers are no larger than an 'o' on this page, they would be impossible to detect by this method. As they grow larger, they are more easily detectable. Gently feel the breast for lumps or thickenings. Be especially aware of the area between the nipple and the armpit because this is a common place for cancerous lumps to occur. In addition to this test, you can examine the breast while showering or bathing because the skin is smoother at this time. Either of these checks will be more effective if done just after the menstrual period because the breasts will have lost some of their fullness.

Report any changes to your doctor. In addition to these self-checks, your doctor should examine you periodically. The doctor may use other diagnostic techniques such as X-ray (mammography), or a test for the heat given off by the breast may be used. Abnormal cancer cells give off more heat than normal cells. A new test, called biofield examination, is being tested. It measures the electrical output of the cells. When it is perfected, it will be more accurate than the mammogram.

Mammograms, low-dose X-rays, are recommended for women starting from the age of 40 to 50, depending on their risk factors. Experts are not in agreement yet as to whether 40 is too early begin these checks. A mammogram can detect tumours and cysts which are too small to be detected by the fingers. Mammograms should be scheduled the week after one's menstrual flow because the potential pain caused by squeezing the breasts during the X-ray is reduced when the breasts are smaller and less tender.

There are seven major types of breast cancers and a number of non-cancerous types of breast problems, several of which will show lumps, thickening or pain. For this reason, a woman should stay in close contact with her doctor regarding any breast abnormalities.

Preventative methods for avoiding breast cancer include making certain that you are getting enough vitamin A and exercising effectively. Women who exercised four hours a week from the time they started menstruating reduced their risk by 60 per cent. Those who exercised one to three hours per week reduced their risk by 30 per cent.[6]

Men can also contract breast cancer. Each year, 1,000 men are diagnosed with the disease and 300 will die from it.

LUNG CANCER

Lung cancer takes many lives each year. Its frequency is increasing greater than any other cancer. (There are more than twenty different cancer-producing ingredients in cigarettes and cigarette smoke.) Every 7 minutes someone dies of lung cancer. It cannot be determined by X-rays until it has passed beyond the curable stage. It therefore must be prevented since it cannot be effectively diagnosed and cured early.

If you are a smoker, your chances of contracting lung cancer are: eight times greater than non-smokers if you smoke half a pack a day; nine times greater if you smoke one half to one pack a day; ten times greater if you smoke one to two packs; and twenty times greater if you smoke more than two packs a day. One marijuana joint contains the same amount of cancer-producing agents as twenty cigarettes.

CANCER OF THE LOWER INTESTINE

Cancer of the lower intestine accounts for over 150,000 cases each year and about 57,000 deaths each year. Genetic factors may be responsible for as many as one in seven cases. When detected early, this cancer is over 80 per cent curable.

The type of food we eat may be an important factor in determining whether or not we develop cancer of the intestines. Recent studies have indicated that high-fibre diets may move the food through the intestines quicker, which may explain why there appears to be a lower incidence of intestinal cancer among people who are on a high fibre diet. Beer drinking may be a negative factor. Studies have shown a range of 50 per cent to 300 per cent increase in this cancer among beer drinkers as opposed to non-drinkers.

There is now a test to check for inherited factors which contribute to colon cancer; 15 per cent of colon cancers are related to a recently discovered gene. For most people, a simple test that checks for blood in the stools is used. Of every thousand people tested for such blood, one hundred will have blood in their stools. Of these, only three will have colon cancer.

DETECTING CANCER

The seven danger signals of cancer are:

- Changes in bowel or bladder habits.
- A sore that does not heal.
- Unusual bleeding or discharge.
- Thickening or lump in the breasts or elsewhere.
- Indigestion or difficulty in swallowing.
- Obvious change in a wart or mole.
- Nagging cough or hoarseness.

Nearly one-third of those who will die of cancer this year could have been cured if the disease had been diagnosed early. If people are aware of the seven danger signals of cancer and have the appropriate tests done by

---

Most Common Signs for Skin Cancer

- An open sore which takes at least three weeks to heal.
- A reddish patch anywhere on the body.
- A smooth circular growth with a raised edge and a depressed centre.
- A shiny reddish or milky coloured bump.
- A pale mark that looks like a scar.
- A wart that bleeds and scabs.
- A mole which is not circular and small. Normal warts are generally less than a quarter of an inch in diameter.
- A mole of irregular shape or with more than one colour, including white, red, brown, blue or black.
- Moles that feel rough, itch or hurt.
- The skin around a mole that is grey, white, red or swollen.

---

physicians, their chances of early diagnosis and longer life would be greatly increased.

There *are* tests that can be medically performed to determine whether or not a person has cancer:

- The previously-mentioned annual medical examinations and the self-tests of the breast can be the most important. Mammograms for breasts and Pap smears for cervical cancer are essential.
- The proctoscopy is effective for finding cancer of the colon and the rectum.
- The barium enema combined with an X-ray may show abnormalities of the large intestine.
- A test to discover if there is blood in the faeces is a method of determining colon cancer.
- The upper digestive tract can be checked by swallowing a barium solution and X-raying it as it passes through the body.
- Leukaemia can be determined by taking a white blood-cell count.

• Cancer of the urinary tract can be detected by checking for blood cells in the urine. It has been found that, by using two different types of dyes, the malignant cells, especially those found in bladder cancers, have a strong attraction to one of the stains and become deeply pigmented before the healthy cells do. This can indicate bladder cancer long before the normal methods would be able to find it.

REDUCING YOUR CHANCES OF CONTRACTING CANCERS

Nearly all of the well-known rules for maintaining health assist in preventing cancers and other diseases: avoid tobacco and marijuana; if you drink, do it moderately; exercise; eat effectively, making certain that you get enough of the vegetables containing beta carotene and fibres; keep your fat intakes low; control your weight; and avoid the sun.

Cancer Survival Rates Following Treatment

Among those cancers which have been discovered early and treated, the 5-year survival rates are as follows:

	If the cancer was localized	If the cancer had spread to other areas
Breast	82%	47%
Colon and rectal	68%	34%
Lung	21%	5%
Mouth	53%	13%
Skin	92%	no regional involvement
Uterus	91%	46%

These figures indicate the extreme importance of early diagnosis and treatment.

CHAPTER 5
Other Chronic and Degenerative Diseases

ARTHRITIS

Arthritis (inflammation of the joints) is a major crippler, affecting millions of people. Half of the people over 65 have some type of arthritis. There are really about one hundred types of arthritis, of which the major categories are:

- Traumatic arthritis, which is due to injury;
- Osteoarthritis, caused by the normal wear and tear of ageing;
- Rheumatoid arthritis, which is apparently the result of an anti-immune reaction;
- Gout, which is caused by the build-up of uric acid in the joints.

Traumatic arthritis can result from injuries such as sports injuries. Some tennis elbows and football or basketball knees are such examples. Car accidents can cause whip lashes that result in arthritis conditions in the neck.

Osteoarthritis is the most common, affecting millions of people, usually those over 50. There is a strong hereditary link, although some sports activities can speed up the process. Some 'tennis elbow' conditions or 'swimmer's shoulders' result from overuse and earlier ageing. Joint replacement, particularly hips and knees, is often used to correct this condition. Moderate, low-impact exercise such as walking, swimming or cycling has been shown to reduce symptoms while increasing fitness.[1]

Rheumatoid arthritis is classified as an auto-immune disease because a substance called 'the rheumatoid factor', which is an antibody, reacts against one of the blood proteins (gamma globulin). There is evidence, however, that rheumatoid arthritis might also be caused by a type of bacteria – Type B streptococcus. This germ is found in the nose and mouth of about 80 per cent of people with rheumatoid arthritis, but only about 20 per cent of the people without the disease. It has also been hypothesized that this bacterium can be transmitted in milk because it is one of the few bacteria to withstand the temperatures of pasteurization. Because the disease is carried through the blood, all of the body's joints may be infected. Some rheumatoid-type conditions are caused by a reaction to streptococcus such as in rheumatic fever or to gonorrhoeal infections.

Gout is another type of arthritis, most often attacking middle-aged men. It is caused by a build-up of uric acid in the joints. A change in diet, limiting certain kinds of proteins such as are found in liver, and the reduction or elimination of alcohol from the diet are most commonly recommended. Drugs can also be used to reduce the uric acid concentration.

Doctors cannot currently cure arthritis, but they can often reduce the severity of the disease and the disability and deformities caused by it. Through drugs, proper exercise, surgery, physical therapy and other treatments, many arthritic patients can be helped. Generally, a change of climate or a change of diet does not help an arthritic patient. Gout is an exception.

All that can be done is to decrease the perception of the pain. This is why aspirin often works, because its analgesic properties make people less aware of the pain that is caused by their ailment. However, acetaminophen (Tylenol) is generally recommended as the first type of treatment, especially for osteoarthritis.[2]

- Maintain good posture (lift with your legs not your back, sit up, don't slouch.)
- If surgery is suggested, get a second opinion.

Keeping the back flexible and strong is essential in order to reduce the possibility of lower back strain and sprain.

BACK PAIN

Back pain is the second most frequent reason for people visiting the doctor (having a cold is the most frequent). Huge amounts of money are spent on treatment and operations. However, many operations do not help. The common diagnostic tool, magnetic resonance imaging (MRI), will often find an abnormality in the spinal column, but such abnormalities may not be the cause of the problem. In one study, 66 per cent of people with no lower back pain were shown to have abnormalities in their spines.[3]

Suggested treatment of lower back pain initially is:

- One or two days of bed rest – no more.
- Non-prescription painkillers such as aspirin.
- Walk, swim or ride a bicycle exerciser as soon as possible.
- If riding a bike, adjust the seat and handlebars so that you can sit upright, not lean forward.
- Do the proper lower back stretches and strength exercises. (*See* the appropriate chapters.)
- Always warm up before back exercises by walking or doing gentle callisthenics. Applying warmth before an exercise and cold afterwards can help to reduce any pain.
- When stretching, stretch slowly and hold.
- Sometimes chiropractic treatment is helpful.
- Do not use traction.
- Do not smoke.

CHRONIC FATIGUE SYNDROME

As the name implies, this is a feeling of tiredness that is nearly continual. It is generally also accompanied by sleep disturbances and muscle and joint pains. It has only recently been officially recognized as a disease. It is most likely linked to immune system problems and perhaps a viral infection. Because so little is known about its causes, it is difficult to diagnose accurately. For this reason, the estimates of its incidence range from between 10,000 to five million people. About 85 per cent of those affected are women.

DiABETES

Diabetes is the seventh major cause of death. Hispanics have about double the risk of other population groups.[4] Diabetes affects the pancreas, causing a deficiency of insulin which metabolizes sugar. The symptoms of diabetes include: excessive thirst, increased output of urine, unusual weight loss and fatigue. It is the number one cause of blindness.

There are two general types of diabetes. Type I or non-insulin-dependent diabetes mellitus (NIDDM), previously called juvenile onset diabetes, occurs when the body is not able to manufacture insulin to metabolize the blood sugar. About 10 per cent of diabetics have this form of the disease. Type II or insulin-dependent diabetes mellitus (IDDM), formerly called maturity onset diabetes, occurs when the amount of insulin produced is insufficient for the diabetic, or the cells become resistant to using it. This type is more likely to develop after the age of 40.

Type II often happens to overweight people, even overweight children. Quite often by controlling their diet and possibly by giving them insulin, this can be controlled. Type I diabetes, while more common in the young, can occur in very old people. Similarly, type II can occur in young people, although it is more likely to start when we are older.

There are many people who have the disease without knowing it. Since diet and exercise play a big part in type II diabetes, people who live healthily may not develop any symptoms. In a study of 20,000 physicians, exercising once a week reduced the incidence of diabetes by 28 per cent, exercising two to four times a week by 38 per cent.[4]

Diabetes is hereditary, although it can be brought on more rapidly by environmental factors such as being overweight or by a lack of exercise. About 75 per cent of people with type II diabetes are obese, that is, at least 20 per cent overweight. As a hereditary disease it is estimated that about 45 million people carry the genetic capability to transmit it.

Diabetics have a much higher than normal risk of heart disease. This is thought to be due to a number of factors: the rate at which some white blood cells bind to the artery walls thus leading to atherosclerosis; a reduced ability to dissolve blood clots because of an excess of a blood element which can increase clotting; and, for women, an increase in the amount of LDL (bad) cholesterol.[5]

EMPHYSEMA

This is another chronic disease, affecting many millions of people, usually men over 40. Its annual death toll is about 10,000. Emphysema often results from cigarette smoking, asthma or chronic bronchitis. It is a result of the breakdown of the small air sacs of the lungs. When these sacs break, the oxygen exchange cannot take place as easily.

The victim of emphysema may breathe twenty to thirty times per minute (fourteen is normal), but still, the oxygen will not be sufficient. Other symptoms of emphysema are shortness of breath, a heavy cough and, often, a feeling of choking. The chances of developing emphysema are increased if the person is a smoker, breathes through the mouth or breathes dirty air.

FIBROMYALALGIA

Fibromyalalgia is an arthritis-like condition which affects the connective tissues – tendons (which connect bones to muscles) and ligaments (which connect bones to other bones). It affects six million people, with women afflicted ten times more often than men. It is also more likely to attack those over 50, although it can affect people as early as in their twenties. In addition to the localized pain, which can occur in any joint or in the upper rib areas of the chest or back, there may be general fatigue, headaches, abdominal pain, constipation or diarrhoea, and a sensitivity to temperature changes. Sleep disorders, particularly a poor deep resting phase of sleep (delta or phase IV) and poor physical fitness are also effects of this disease.

Although the symptoms have been around for many years and labelled a number of different ways, the disease has only recently been named and its symptoms recognized. It was added to the World Health Organization's list of diseases only in 1992. Previously it had been diagnosed as flu, arthritis, ageing problems, Lyme disease or other maladies which created joint pain.

HEADACHES

These affect nearly half of us. Forty million people experience them with sufficient severity to ask for medical assistance. About ten million people suffer from migraines, which are very severe forms of headache. Most headache sufferers are women, but men tend to have more severe headaches.

A headache is not really a disease, but rather a symptom of disease. It can be a symptom of very severe physical problems, such as brain tumours. It can be caused by hormonal problems, or can be a symptom of allergies. Migraines are often triggered by odours or foods. Stress can also cause a migraine.

It appears now that there is probably a single underlying mechanism for most or all headaches.[6] However, there are several types of headaches:

- The vascular (blood vessel) type occurs when the arteries both inside and outside of the scalp are dilated and engorged with blood. The enlargement of the arteries then pushes against the nerves and pain is experienced. The pain may be a throbbing corresponding to the pulse rate. All migraine headaches are of this sort.
- A 'hang-over' headache is also the result of dilation and the distention of the blood vessels of the scalp which push on the nerve centres and cause pain.
- Headaches can also be muscular. These are usually located at the base of the skull.
- Tension headaches may be related to muscle contraction or fatigue and are very often brought on by emotional pressure or depression. Many people seem to feel the need to have everything very orderly, putting a great amount of pressure on themselves. This can lead to headaches of this type.
- Depression headaches often occur on weekends, holidays, the first day of a holiday, or the first day after examinations. People who suffer from these headaches are often first children. They may be angry at loved ones and not realize it.
- Pressure headaches occur when pain-sensitive structures on the inside or outside of the skull are stimulated. These can be due to tumours or other types of growth abnormalities.
- Inflammation headaches can occur when pain-sensitive structures are stimulated by an infection or another source of inflammation.

About half of the people who suffer from headaches have the vascular blood vessel headaches. These include migraine sufferers and the cluster headache sufferers. Other headaches are emotional or psychogenic in origin. These are usually caused by depression and tension. About 47 per cent of headache sufferers have these.

Some headaches are the result of allergies. Among the foods which commonly cause these allergies are chocolate, some dairy products, some cheeses, onions, citrus fruits, pork, seafood, fried foods, hot dogs and dried food. Alcohol and tobacco can also contribute to this kind of headache.

Monosodium glutamate, a flavour enhancer frequently used in Chinese cooking, also can bring on headaches, as can sodium nitrite, which is found in sausages. Of the foods which tend to elicit headaches, they seem to all have a type of amino acid (tyrosine), which is important in the transmission of nervous impulses. When the headache sufferer does not have the enzyme necessary to metabolize these substances, a headache occurs. A prevailing theory is that an area of the hypothalamus, which is located in the brain and which controls the constriction and dilation of the blood vessels, may be stimulated by the allergies when the necessary enzyme is not present to metabolize the substances to which the person is allergic.

Cold can also elicit headaches. Of adult migraine victims, 93 per cent suffer 'ice-cream headache' – whenever they bite into something cold, they get a strong pain. Only 31 per cent of the people who do not get headaches have such a reaction.

Many doctors have shown that some vascular headaches such as migraines are often relieved by getting blood away from the head and into another part of the body, such as the hands. This reduces the distension of the blood vessels which causes this type of headache. Hand warming can be done by putting them into warm water or by using biofeedback. This technique does not work on other types of headaches such as tension headaches.

Other things which might relieve headache symptoms are aspirin (as an analgesic), coffee (which may stimulate other blood vessels to open), exercise (which puts blood into other areas of the body than the brain), fresh air, and drugs which constrict the blood vessel. Stress-reducing activities can also be valuable when the cause of the headache is stress-related. New drugs are also being developed to control the neurotransmitters, such as serotonin, which are often related to the physical causes of the blood-vessel changes in the brain.

KIDNEY STONES

These are developed when people eat certain types of foods, especially those containing oxalic acid such as spinach and rhubarb. High levels of vitamin C can also cause kidney stones, generally because of the binding agents in the pill. The chances of developing such stones are decreased by drinking a great deal of water, at least a glass in the morning and glass before every meal, and preferably eight glasses a day.

OSTEOPOROSIS

Osteoporosis (porous bones) is a condition which is most often found in post-menopausal women, particularly those with smaller bones. Due to a lack of oestrogen (because of the menopause, a lack of calcium in the diet, or a lack of weight-bearing activities) the bones begin to lose their structure. In some people, this shows as an extreme curvature of the upper back, due to the loss of bone in the vertebrae in the neck and thoracic areas, which forces the head downward. More commonly, it is seen in the thinning of the upper part of the thigh bone. Most of the broken hips experienced by older people are caused by this bone loss. People think that they fell, then their hip broke, in fact, in most cases the hip actually broke first, as weight was put on it, then the person fell.

Bones are active tissues, giving off and replacing calcium continually. At about age 35 women's bones begin to become less dense. This happens a little later for men. After menopause, female bone loss is increased because of the lack of oestrogen. By age 65, the average woman has lost 26 per cent of her bone density, while the average man has lost 9 per cent. The best methods of reducing the risk are:

- A lifelong intake of calcium (preferably non-fat milk or cheese) and/or calcium supplements. While the normal recommended daily intake of calcium is 800 to 1,000mg, many experts suggest that post-menopausal women should take 1,500mg daily.[7]
- Weight-bearing exercise (dancing, gardening, housework, walking, running, and so on – yoga and swimming do not qualify).
- Do not smoke.
- If you drink, drink in moderation.
- For post-menopausal women, hormone replacement therapy is often a possibility.

45

Heredity plays a part in the potential for developing the condition. Small-boned people, particularly Asians and Caucasians, are at risk. Black women seem to have higher bone density, so are less at risk. If you haven't been consuming enough calcium and vitamin D, you can rebuild bone to some degree and reduce your chances of fracturing your bones, particularly breaking your hip, by supplementing these nutrients.

In a major study over a three-year period using men and women 65 years of age or older, dietary supplementation with calcium and vitamin D moderately reduced bone loss measured in the femoral neck, spine and total body during the study period and reduced the incidence of non-vertebral fractures. The people in the study received 500mg of calcium plus 700 IU of vitamin D^3 (cholecalciferol) per day.

VARICOSE VEINS

These affect many people, particularly women. When the veins are under greater pressure from the blood, the valves which prevent the blood from moving downwards may be swollen. As the valves swell, the veins appear to bulge. This can occur because the veins are close to the skin or because they do not have enough support from the muscles. Varicose veins may occur in people who are very muscular, or in women who are pregnant because the pressure of the uterus makes it more difficult for the blood to pass through the abdominal area, so creating additional pressure on the valves of the veins.

In many cases, the tendency towards varicose veins is inherited. Weak or malformed valves in the veins could be inherited. Environmental factors can also contribute to varicose veins. People who are overweight or do heavy lifting will often have varicose veins.

In order to prevent or slow the occurrence of varicose veins, it would be best to exercise, walk or swim, but do not stand or even sit down for too long. Good muscle activity will help to massage the blood back through the veins and towards the heart. You can also elevate your feet occasionally so that the blood has gravity assisting it in its flow towards the heart. If the varicose veins are very large, it is possible for physicians to operate or to use injections to minimize the pain and also their unsightliness.

INTERNET SOURCES OF INFORMATION

http://ntserver.ih2000.net/osteoporosis/ Osteoporosis Online from Southeast Texas University
http://www.nof.org/ National Osteoporosis Foundation
http://www.lookup.com/Homepages/55273/home.html Osteoporosis Society of British Columbia (Local resources for this Canadian province as well as a summary of the disease.)

CHAPTER 6
Protein, Fats and Carbohydrates

This chapter deals with the basic nutrients which we must consume. The next three chapters will deal with vitamins and minerals, the types of foods we eat and some things that we should consider in relation to our eating habits and managing our weight, as well as some recent research on supplementing our diets. While we must obtain our nutrients, we also may be interested in taste, our weight and other elements that we, in the twentieth century, have found to be both delights and problems.

As we age, our nutritional needs may change. We need fewer calories to maintain our weight. Our diets may become less nutritious, yet our bodies may need higher levels of some nutrients to ward off diseases. So we must be aware of what is needed and how to get what we need.

NUTRITION

A basic understanding of the science of nutrition is essential to healthy living. An informed person will be aware of the nutrients that are necessary for minimal functioning, then put that knowledge into practice by developing a proper diet. Unfortunately, very few people consume even the minimum amounts of all nutrients. Their diets may be lacking in protein, fat, carbohydrates, vitamins, minerals, fibre, or water (the essential non-nutrient).

The first three nutrients listed (protein, fat and carbohydrates) bring with them the energy required to keep us alive, in addition to their specific contributions to the body that will be discussed in detail later. All of the food energy that we consume comes in the form of calories. The last three nutrients (vitamins, minerals and fibre) do not bring with them calories when consumed.

The Calorie

The calorie used in counting food energy is really a kilocalorie, one thousand times larger than the calorie commonly used as a measurement of heat in chemistry classes. In one food calorie (kilocalorie), there is enough energy to heat 1kg (2.2lb) of water 1 to degree Celsius, or to lift 3,000lb (1,360kg) of weight 1ft (30cm) high. So those little calories that you see listed on the biscuit box pack a lot of energy!

In the more scientific literature, food energy is often listed in terms of joules or kilojoules (kJ). The joule is a measure of work rather than a measure of heat. To convert a kilocalorie into its kilojoule equivalent multiply it by 4.2. In this book, we will use the measure of calories since it is still commonly used by most people.

Most people need about 10 calories per pound (500g) just to stay alive. If you plan to do something other than just lie in bed all day, you may need about 17 calories per pound of body weight per day in order to keep yourself going. The starvation level for the average person is around 1,300 calories per day.

PROTEIN

Protein is made up of twenty-two amino acids, otherwise known as the 'building blocks of life'. Amino acids are made up of carbon, hydrogen, oxygen and nitrogen. While both fats and carbohydrates contain the first three elements, nitrogen is found only in protein. Protein is essential for building nearly every part of the body – the brain, heart, organs, skin, muscles and even the blood.

There are 4 calories in 1g of protein, although there are measures indicating that it is 5.6 calories. Adults require 0.75g of protein per kilogram of body weight per day, unless their particular body utilizes more protein, as is the case with muscular dystrophy patients. This translates into one-third of a gram of protein per pound of body weight. So, an easy estimate for your protein requirements in grams per day would be to divide your body weight in pounds by 3. For instance, if you weigh 150lb (68kg), you need about 50g of protein per day. The elderly may require as much protein per day as do children (1.15g per kg per day) due to their decreased energy intake coupled by a possible decreased utilization of dietary protein

Physically active adults have been thought to require more protein than is recommended by the Recommended Daily Allowance (RDA), which is set at 0.8 grams per kilogram of body weight per day. In fact, most active people need not eat additional protein if they consume to 12–15 per cent of their total calories as protein. Since active individuals need to consume more calories per day than their inactive counterparts due to their increased energy expenditure, active adults who keep their protein intake at around 15 per cent of their total calories will eat more protein per day and thereby fulfil their body's protein requirement.[1] Excess protein consumption (above the body's requirement) will be broken down and the calories will either be burned off or stored as fat.

However, when involved in a strenuous strength-training regimen, it may be necessary to increase your protein intake percentage depending on the amount of total calories you consume per day. Strength-trained athletes have been shown to adapt to diets considered low in protein (0.86 grams per kilogram per day) by decreasing their overall body protein synthesis. This is not a good idea since the purpose of strength training is to build muscle, and you don't want to do anything to hamper this process. Therefore, those who participate in heavy resistance training may choose to follow a diet that is higher in protein (1.4g per kilogram per day) to elicit maximum benefits from their workout.[2] This increased protein demand also appears true for novice body-builders who trained intensively (1.5 hours per day, 6 days per week) for one month.[3]

In order to create anything in your body, including muscle, you must first have all of the necessary amino acids. Some of them your body can manufacture, while others you must get from your food. Those amino acids that you must get from your food are called the essential amino acids, while the others that you can make are known as the non-essential amino acids. During childhood, nine of the twenty-two amino acids are essential, while in adulthood we acquire the ability to synthesize one additional amino acid, leaving us with eight essential amino acids.

Amino acids cannot be stored in the body. People therefore need to consume their minimum amounts of protein every day. If adequate protein is not consumed, the body immediately begins to break down tissue (usually beginning with muscle tissue) to release the essential amino acids. If even one essential amino acid is lacking, the other essential ones are not able to work to their full capacities.

For example, if methionine (the most commonly lacking amino acid) is present at 60 per cent of the minimum requirement, the other seven essential amino acids are limited to nearly 60 per cent of their potential. When they are not used, amino acids are deaminated and excreted as urea in the urine.

Animal products (fish, poultry and beef) and animal by-products (milk, eggs and cheese) are rich in readily usable protein. This means that when you eat animal products or by-products, the protein you consume can be converted into protein in your body because these sources have all of the essential amino acids in them. These foods are called complete protein sources.

Essential Amino Acids and Foods in which they are Found

- *Iso-leucine:* fish, beef, organ meats, eggs, shellfish, whole wheat, soya, milk.
- *Leucine:* beef, fish, organ meats, eggs, soya, shellfish, whole wheat, milk, liver.
- *Lysine:* fish, beef, organ meats, shellfish, eggs, soya, milk, liver.
- *Methionine:* fish, beef, shellfish, eggs, milk, liver, whole wheat, cheese.
- *Phenylalanine:* beef, fish, eggs, whole wheat, shellfish, organ meats, soya, milk.
- *Threonine:* fish, beef, organ meats, eggs, shellfish, soya, liver.
- *Tryptophan:* soya milk, fish, beef, soy flour, organ meats, shell fish, eggs.
- *Valine:* beef, fish, organ meats, eggs, soya, milk, whole wheat, liver.
- *Cystine* (sis'ten) is a non-essential amino acid that can be ingested or made from methionine; thus, the two are often listed together.

Incomplete protein sources are any other food sources that provide protein, but not all of the essential amino acids. Some examples of incomplete proteins include beans, peas and nuts. These food sources must be combined with other food sources that have the missing essential amino acids so that you can make protein in your body. Some examples of complementary foods are rice and beans, or peanut butter on whole-wheat bread.

Being aware of specific food combinations can help to enhance the absorption of the protein that has been consumed. For example, if flour is eaten at breakfast (such as a piece of toast or coffee cake) and washed down with coffee, and then a glass of milk is consumed at lunch, each of the protein sources would be absorbed by the body at a lower potential. But if the bread was consumed with milk at either meal, the higher protein values of both would be absorbed by the body immediately.

Not all protein sources are equally good. The most common protein foods were ranked according to protein quality by the Food and Agricultural Organization of the United

---

Most Common Protein Foods[4]

The higher the rating, the better the essential amino-acid ratio – that is, more of the essential amino acids are present. According to the ranking:

	Biological value	Amino-acid score
Whole eggs	94%	100%
Cow's milk	84%	98%
Fish	83%	100%
Beef	74%	100%
Soya beans	73%	63%
Brown rice	73%	59%
White potatoes	67%	48%
Whole-grain wheat	65%	45%
Beans	58%	46%
Peanuts	54%	55%

	Lysine (mg)	Methionine (and cystine)(mg)	Tryptophan (mg)
Hen's egg	167	138	107
Cow's milk	169	79	100
Soya beans	167	67	100
White wheat flour	55	105	86
Mixture of ⅓ milk and ⅔ flour	93	95	93
Mixture of ⅓ soy-bean and ⅔ flour	93	93	93

Nations in 1957 and revised in 1973.[4] The higher the rating, the better the essential amino-acid ratio – that is, more of the essential amino acids are present. According to the ranking, whole eggs have the highest quality of protein with a ranking of 94 per cent (its biological rating). Cow's milk is second with a biological rating of 84 per cent; fish rates an 83 per cent rating and beef 74 per cent.

In 1972, the Food and Agricultural Organization refined their findings by rating the quantity of each amino acid in a food. Above is an example of the rankings based on the percentages of three of the essential amino acids (*see* box above).

From the chart, you can see that even the highly rated milk or soya beans are relatively low in methionine and cystine. But if we combined them with wheat flour, we can bring their protein quality into the 93 to 95 range. And the flour, which rated 86 per cent in tryptophan, was raised to 93 per cent.

It should be noted that in eggs 56 per cent of the protein and 20 per cent of the calories are in the egg white, while all of the fat and cholesterol are in the egg yolk. Similarly, skimmed milk actually yields more protein than whole milk at only half of the calories with no fat.

Protein Supplements

These are used by some people, particularly weight trainers and athletes. They may be dangerous. Infants under one year of age and older people with liver or kidney ailments often cannot handle the highly concentrated doses of protein contained in these commercially prepared supplements. Also they usually fall far short of a good balance of the essential amino acids. While six of the essential amino acids are usually present in good quantities in these supplements, methionine and tryptophan are usually found in lesser amounts. Since 910mg of methionine and 245mg of tryptophan are the recommended daily allowances, you might check to determine how much of these are actually contained in a supplement. This is especially important if your diet is lacking in either one or both of these amino acids and you are primarily relying on the supplement to account for most or all of your protein needs. A better and cheaper source of protein for one needing a supplement would be powdered milk. If your diet is deficient in protein, you might consider using egg whites (or egg substitutes), milk, fish or chicken. It may prove less expensive and more nutritious.

FAT

Fat consists of carbon, hydrogen and oxygen. There are 9.4 calories in a gram of fat. In the body, fat is used to develop the myelin sheath that surrounds the nerves. It also aids in the absorption of vitamins A, D, E and K, which are the fat-soluble vitamins. It serves as a protective layer around our vital organs, and is an insulator against the cold. It is also an outstanding concentrated energy source. And, of course, its most redeeming quality is that it adds flavour and juiciness to food!

Just as protein is broken down into different kinds of nitrogen compounds called amino acids, there are also different kinds of fats. There are three major fats (fatty acids): saturated fats, monounsaturated fats and polyunsaturated fats.

Saturated fats are 'saturated' with hydrogen atoms. They are generally solid at room temperature and are most likely found in animal fats, egg yolks and the cream in whole milk products. Since these are the fats that are primarily responsible for raising the blood cholesterol level and hardening the arteries, they should be minimized.

Monounsaturated fats (oleic fatty acids) have room for two hydrogen ions to double bond to one carbon. They are liquid at room temperature and are found in great amounts in olive, peanut and rapeseed oils. Dietary monounsaturated fats have been shown to have the greatest effect on the efflux of cholesterol, thereby reducing the tendency of the arteries to harden.[5]

Polyunsaturated fats (linoleic fatty acids) have at least two carbon double bonds available, which translates into space for at least four hydrogen ions. Polyunsaturated fats are also liquid at room temperature and are found in the highest proportions in vegetable sources. Safflower, corn and linseed oils are good sources of this type of fat. Polyunsaturated fatty acids of the Omega-3 type may also contribute to the prevention of atherosclerosis.[6] However, this seems to be specific to the consumption of actual fish rather than fish oil pills. In addition, some studies suggest that dietary polyunsaturated fats, when consumed in large amounts, may have a harmful effect on atherosclerosis if they are not eaten with adequate antioxidants.[7] The antioxidants will be covered later.

Just as the percentage of each amino acid varies in different types of foods, the amounts and percentages of the different types of fats vary from food to food.

We eat too much fat. The minimum requirement for fat in the diet is considered to be somewhere between 10 and 20 per cent of the total calories consumed. The absolute maximum should be 30 per cent, which is the amount now recommended for the Western diet. While we, as a society, are still above this 30 per cent value, our consumption has been declining since the 1970s, so let's try to keep that trend going. Most of us consume between 35 and 50 per cent of our total calories in fats. Also, our typical diet is very high in saturated fats, which are the fats that we want to avoid. If we had not been too careful about this in our youth, it is time now to change for the better.

Our high fat intake, most of which is saturated, tends to raise blood cholesterol levels in many people. For those who wish to lower their blood cholesterol level, a diet low in fat is recommended (with the saturated fat intake at 10 per cent or less of the total diet), combined with an intake of less than 300mg of cholesterol daily. Put another way, keep the total calories from fat to under a third of your total intake and eat twice as much polyunsaturated and monounsaturated fats as saturated fat.

A recent study, which summarized a large number of studies, indicated that 'in typical British diets replacing 60 per cent of saturated fats by other fats and avoiding 60 per cent of dietary cholesterol would reduce blood total cholesterol by about 0.8 mmol/l (that is, by 10–15 per cent), with four-fifths of this reduction being in low density lipoprotein cholesterol.' The latter is the 'bad' cholesterol.[8]

In the past, companies were allowed to identify the oil in a product on their labels merely as vegetable oil; under more recent requirements, they must now note whether it is corn oil, cottonseed oil, soya bean oil, and so on, because some of the oils, even though they are not of animal origin, are very high in saturated fat. Palm kernel oil and coconut oil are particularly high in saturated fats. Some countries are still allowed to state on their food packages that the product contains one of several oils such as: 'contains one of the following oils: rapeseed, soya, or palm kernel oil'. When this listing occurs, you can be fairly sure that the oil is the harmful palm kernel oil – the others are more expensive.

As can be seen from the previous chart, corn oil or safflower oil margarines are far better than butter in terms of the ratio of polyunsaturated to saturated fats. Butter has 17g of saturated fat to one gram of polyunsaturated fat, while safflower margarine has one gram of saturated fat to 2.5g of polyunsaturated fat. The margarine is obviously far better in terms of its ratio of fat, but both margarine and butter contribute to the total fat intake. In addition, in order to make margarine stay solid at room temperature, hydrogen gas has been bubbled through the oil to chemically saturate the open bonds. This then leaves you with a chemically saturated polyunsaturated fat! The harder the margarine, the more it has been through the hydrogenation process and the more chemically saturated polyunsaturated fats you have in the margarine. The result of this is that your blood trans-fatty acid levels increase with the consumption of this type of fat, and the risks of this are still being explored. So, while we know that saturated fat increases blood cholesterol which, in turn, increases your risk of heart disease, the consumption of margarine may also be a risk factor in heart disease and cancers due to the trans-fatty acids.

When buying foods, especially biscuits and crackers, always check the type of fat used. Avoid those with palm kernel oil and coconut oil. Also be aware of the hydrogenated oils that have been used. While a hydrogenated safflower or rapeseed oil may still have an acceptable fat ratio, a hydrogenated peanut or cottonseed oil may not. Partially hydrogenated vegetable oils may contribute to the development of heart disease.[9] The dietary use of hydrogenated corn oil stick margarine increased LDL cholesterol levels when compared to the use of similar amounts of corn oil, also indicating an increased risk of heart disease through the use of hydrogenation.[10]

Eggs, which are another staple in the average diet, contain a great deal of cholesterol and saturated fat in the yolk. The American Heart Association suggests that no more than four egg yolks be eaten per week. This includes egg yolks that are hidden in other foods, such as cakes, custards, some bread, noodles and waffles. An egg yolk contains nearly 300mg of cholesterol, which is the recommended daily *maximum* for cholesterol intake. In addition, the saturated fat in the yolk contributes to one's blood cholesterol profile in a negative way. So, while the egg white is a good source of protein in the diet, the egg yolk is something to be avoided.

In order to allow us to have our scrambled eggs without contributing to our risk of heart disease, some companies have developed a low-cholesterol egg substitute. Since most of the cholesterol is found in the yolks of the eggs, they have removed the yolk and substituted corn oil, non-fat dry milk and other additives. This drops the cholesterol level of one egg from 275mg to less than one milligram of cholesterol. The egg substitute can also be used in cooking. Egg substitutes can be found in the frozen food or egg sections at the market. If you do your own baking it is recommended that rather than using a whole egg in a recipe, use an egg substitute or replace one egg with two egg whites and throw away the yolks.

Whole milk, another diet staple, contains 3.5 per cent fat, accounting for nearly half of its total calories. Semi-skimmed milk has between 1 and 2 per cent fat. Whole milk contains 320 calories from fat per quart and low-fat milk contains about 184 calories from fat per quart, while skimmed milk has minimal, if any, fat. But each type of milk contains about the same amount of protein (145 calories from protein and 200 calories from carbohydrates). So skimmed milk is obviously far superior as a high-protein, low-calorie, no fat-food.

Cholesterol in the diet is not as important as saturated fats in terms of controlling one's blood cholesterol level. For this reason, saturated fats should be reduced. This means that the major sources of saturated fats (red meats, butter, egg yolks, chicken skin and other animal fats) should be greatly decreased. As an informed consumer you may want to keep track of both your total fat intake and your intake of saturated fat to become better aware of your potential risk of heart disease. For example, one egg contains 5.6g of fat and only 0.7g of polyunsaturated fat but 275mg of cholesterol, while an equal weight of ground beef contains 8.7g of fat and only 0.4g of polyunsaturated fats and 45mg of cholesterol.

It may be possible to reverse the build-up of fat in the arteries through a diet that is very low in fat. Experiments with monkeys have shown that the artery plaque could be developed by a high saturated fat diet, but when the monkeys were given a low-fat, low-cholesterol diet for 18 months, 50 per cent of the plaque build-up disappeared. After results from these studies were made public, human studies began, which found that though a very low-fat diet or through medication and diet modification, arterial plaque build-up could be reversed.[11] However, if the build-up has become 'calcified', which often occurs with advancing age, it cannot be reduced.

CARBOHYDRATES

Carbohydrates are made from carbon, hydrogen and oxygen, just like fats, but they are generally a simpler type of molecule. There are four calories in a gram of carbohydrate. If not utilized immediately for energy as sugar (glucose), they are either stored in the body as a sugar called glycogen (the stored form of glucose) or synthesized into fat and stored. Some carbohydrates cannot be broken down by the body's digestive processes. These are called fibres and will be discussed later. Of the digestible carbohydrates, we will separate them into two categories: simple and complex. Simple carbohydrates are the most readily usable energy source in the body and include such things as sugar, honey and fruit. Complex carbohydrates are the starches. These also break down into sugar for energy, but at a slower rate than the simple carbohydrates. Also, complex carbohydrates bring with them various vitamins and minerals.

People often eat too many simple carbohydrates. These are the so-called 'empty calories'. They are empty because they have no vitamins, minerals or fibres. While a person who uses a great deal of energy can consume these empty calories without potential weight gain, most of us find these empty calories settling on our hips. The average person consumes 125lb (57kg) of sugar per year, which is equivalent to one teaspoon every 40 minutes, night and day. Since each teaspoon of sugar contains 17 calories, this amounts to 231,000 calories or 66lb (30kg) of potential body fat if this energy is not used as fuel for daily living.

High-carbohydrate diets that are especially high in sugar may be hazardous to one's health, as they can increase the amount of triglycerides produced in the liver. These triglycerides are blood fats and are possible developers of hardened arteries. Also, a diet high in simple carbohydrates can lead to obesity, which can then result in the development of mature onset diabetes.

Fibre

Fibre is that part of the foods we consume that is not digestible. Fibre helps to move the food through the intestines by increasing their peristaltic action. Vegetable fibres are made up chiefly of cellulose, an indigestible carbohydrate that is the main ingredient in the cell walls of plants. Plant-eating animals, such as cows, can digest cellulose. Meat-eating animals, such as humans, do not have the proper enzymes in their digestive tracts to metabolize cellulose.

Bran (which includes the husks of wheat, oats, rice, rye and corn) is another type of fibre. It is indigestible because of the silica in the outer husks. Some of the fibres, such as wheat bran, are insoluble. Their major function is to add bulk to the faeces and to speed the digested foods through the intestines. This reduces one's risk of constipation, intestinal cancer, appendicitis and diverticulosis.

Diverticulosis is an intestinal problem that is becoming relatively frequent. It is now one of the most common intestinal disorders in Western nations. The diverticulae are pouches similar to small hernias in the intestinal wall. They are caused by either a fold of muscle in the interior wall that pushes outwards, or by a weakness in the internal muscle itself. In either case, the pouch may fill with faecal matter and become infected, resulting in diverticulitis. Experts now believe that these pouches are the final stages of a long-term lack of dietary fibre.

Some types of fibres are soluble; that is, they can pick up certain substances such as dietary cholesterol as they move through the intestines. Pectin, commonly found in raw fruits (especially apple skins), oat and rice brans, and some gums from the seeds and stems of tropical plants (such as guar and xanthin) are examples of soluble fibres.

Foods that are high in fibre are also valuable in weight-reducing diets because they speed the passage of foods through the digestive tract, thereby cutting the amount of possible

Caloric Content of Various Alcoholic Drinks		
Beverages	*Amount*	*Calories*
Ale, 1 bottle	12oz	148
Beer, 1 bottle	12oz	173
Cider, fermented, 1 glass	8oz	73
Daiquiri, 1 glass	6oz	124
Eggnog, 1 punch cup		338
Gin, dry, 1 jigger	1.5oz	107
Manhattan, 1 cocktail		167
Martini, 1 cocktail		143
Whisky, Scotch, 1 glass	1.5oz	107
Wine, red, 1 wine glass		73
Wine, port, 1 wine glass		60

absorption time. They also cut the amount of hunger experienced by a dieter because they fill the stomach. A larger salad with a diet dressing might give the person very few calories but still enough cellulose to fill the stomach, cut the hunger and move other foods through the intestinal passage.

Food processing often removes the natural fibre from the food. This is one of the primary reasons that we have relatively low amounts of fibre in our diet. For instance, white bread has only a trace of fibre – about 9g in a loaf – while old-fashioned whole wheat bread has 70g. Also, when you peel a carrot or an apple, you remove much of the fibre.

Dietitians urge that people include more fibre in their diets, particularly whole-grain cereals, bran and fibrous vegetables. Root vegetables (such as carrots, beets and turnips) and leafy vegetables are very good sources of fibre. The average diet has between 10 to 20g of fibre in it per day, but recommendations to reduce the risk of colon cancer are between 25 to 35g per day.

CHAPTER 7
Vitamins, Minerals and Fibre

Vitamins are organic compounds which are essential in small amounts for the growth and development of animals and humans. They act as enzymes (catalysts) which facilitate many of the body processes. Although there is great controversy regarding the importance of consuming excess vitamins, it is acknowledged that we need a minimum amount of vitamins for proper functioning.

Some vitamins are soluble only in water; others need fat to be absorbed by the body. The water-soluble vitamins, B complex and C, are more fragile than the fat-soluble vitamins. This is because they are more easily destroyed by the heat of cooking and if boiled they lose some of their potency into the water. Since they are not stored by the body, they should be included in the daily diet.

The fat-soluble vitamins, A, D, E and K, need oils in the intestines to be absorbed by the body. They are more stable than the water-soluble vitamins and are not destroyed by normal cooking methods. Because they are stored in the body, there exists the possibility of ingesting too much of them – especially vitamins A and D.

Nutritional researchers disagree as to whether vitamin supplements are necessary. However, they are generally in agreement that natural vitamins are no better than synthetically prepared vitamins. Thus, synthetically-made ascorbic acid *is* vitamin C. There is therefore no need to take rose hips or acerola types of the vitamin in order to get the full effect of vitamin C.

VITAMINS

Vitamin A

Vitamin A is necessary for eyesight as well as skin. During World War II, Denmark began exporting large amounts of butter while supplementing Danish diets with margarine. Many children went blind. It was eventually discovered that the lack of vitamin A in the margarine was responsible for the eye problems. The minimum vitamin A requirements, which the Danes had been consuming when they were eating butter, were reduced when they substituted margarine. Vitamin A was then added to the margarine and no further problems developed.

It is possible to consume too much vitamin A. When this happens, the liver can enlarge, with a resultant loss of appetite or weight, loss of hair, severe bone and joint pain, and cracking lips. It probably requires twenty times the minimum daily requirement over a long period of time before this would occur. A vitamin A overdose case was reported by the US Food and Drug Administration when a woman had taken 75,000 units daily for two years. Among the symptoms she had developed were hair loss, mouth ulcers, extreme fatigue, anaemia, inflammation of the optic nerve and a build-up of pressure within the head that showed the same symptoms as a brain tumour. Recently, a man died from an overdose of vitamin A taken over a long period of time. For this reason, the

US Food and Drug Administration now requires that vitamin A should be limited to 10,000 IU in any non-prescription pill.

Beta carotene is the plant source from which our bodies make vitamin A. Beta carotene does not seem to possess the same toxicity as vitamin A from animal sources. Beta carotene is a powerful antioxidant. Along with other antioxidants, including vitamins C and E, and the mineral selenium, beta carotene 'donates' electrons to free oxygen radicals, making them less destructive.

Free oxygen radicals are harmful substances. They are atoms of oxygen which lack one electron, which makes them unstable. They therefore seek available electrons in other molecules or cells and can cause damage to tissues, or can interfere with the proper chemical reactions in the body. They are believed to be associated with ageing and with about sixty diseases including heart disease, cancers, arthritis, Alzheimer's disease – and even shin splints. They are also suspected of being one of the substances that can start the lesions which develop into atherosclerosis.[1]

They are produced by many natural body processes. Physical exercise, for all of its benefits, is one producer of free oxygen radicals. They are also found in the environment. Air and water pollution, any type of smoke and even dried milk and eggs are some of the environmental sources of these toxins.

Supplementation with antioxidants above the required levels does not appear to increase one's aerobic capacity; however, a deficiency of vitamin C and/or vitamin E has been shown to decrease one's endurance capacity.[2] In addition, the supplementation of antioxidants does not appear to prevent oxidative injury to cells during exercise, but it does appear to help decrease oxidative injury both at rest and after exercise.[3]

In animal and human experiments relating to the effect of the antioxidant properties of vitamins C and E against air pollution and smoke, it was found that vitamin C is more effective in protecting against nitrogen dioxide, while vitamin E is more effective against ozone's oxidative effects. It should be noted, however, that for the maximum protection against the harmful effects of air pollutants, the recommended dietary allowances for both of these vitamins should be increased. Supplementation will be covered in Chapter 9.[4]

The B Vitamins

The B-complex vitamins include at least fifteen substances; only six have been termed essential. The B vitamins seem to work together, particularly in the nervous, circulatory and digestive systems. Some of the B vitamins assist in the break down of proteins, while others help to break down carbohydrates.

Vitamin B1 (thiamin) has been linked with various theories, including a possible link between a thiamin deficiency and Alzheimer's.[5] People consuming abnormally high intakes of alcohol, including those with cirrhosis of the liver, tend to be deficient in thiamin.[6] However, thiamin deficiency can be reversed with supplementation. In a study of elderly people who were initially thiamin-deficient, a thiamin supplement was shown to increase appetite, energy intake, activity, body weight and general wellbeing. In addition, they also showed improved sleep patterns along with reduced sleep requirements during the daytime.[7] There is also some evidence that thiamin in doses of over 5 milligrams a day may act as an insect repellent, since an excess of the vitamin gives the skin an odour that repels some bugs, including mosquitoes.

Vitamin B2 (riboflavin) and vitamin B6 (pyridoxine) deficiencies may prove to hamper one's fitness performance. However, if one is not deficient, there appears to be no additional fitness benefit from further supplementation of these vitamins.[8] With an increase in exercise training, riboflavin requirements have been shown to increase,[9] so it may be important to increase your intake of riboflavin when embarking on or increasing an existing exercise programme. Also, elevated riboflavin levels may provide protection against oxidative damage.[10]

Vitamin B3 (niacin) has been found to inhibit the growth rate of some cancer cells in rats. Pellagra, a niacin deficiency disease, can lead to the development of symptoms of mental illness, such as hallucinations.

Recent research has found that when the body is high in a compound called *homocysteine* there is an increased chance of heart attack. Both folic acid (recommended amounts from 180 to 400 micrograms per day) and vitamin B6 (recommended amount 3mg per day) can reduce the risk significantly.[11]

Vegans, those who consume no animal products or by-products, have diets that are usually deficient in vitamin B12. This is a cause for concern because a vitamin B12 deficiency, in extreme cases, can cause a loss of brain function. Also, a group of vegans in England suffered irreversible destruction of nerve fibres in the spinal cord after 10 to 15 years because of their chronic vitamin B12 deficiency.

Cooking and light can destroy some of the B vitamins. Riboflavin is destroyed very quickly by light and up to 30 per cent may be destroyed in cooking. Milk in a clear bottle, left in the sunlight for two hours, can lose up to 6 per cent of its riboflavin. Thiamin is also destroyed by cooking, especially boiling.[12]

Excessive B vitamins can affect the efficiency of any drugs you may be taking, so it is important to gauge accurately your intake of the B vitamins when taking prescription drugs. For example, riboflavin can interfere with the effects of tetracycline, an antibiotic. Pyridoxine can interfere with levadopa, which is often prescribed for Parkinson's disease. And folic acid can lessen the effects of an antiepileptic drug.

Vitamin C

This is probably the most controversial of all the vitamins, largely because of Linus Pauling's publicity. Vitamin C is claimed by some to have the power to cure sore backs, prevent colds and extend life. These claims are still open to question, but one of the greatest advantages of vitamin C is its antioxidant potential. In a Finnish study reported in the *British Medical Journal*, it was found that men low in vitamin C had a far higher risk of dying from a heart attack than those with normal amounts of the vitamin.[13]

We know that people do need some vitamin C because without 10mg a day, a person would get scurvy – a disease causing weakness and bleeding. In years past, before the effects of vitamin C were understood, whole armies were decimated by scurvy. It is estimated that over 10,000 seamen died in the early days of sea exploration because they did not get enough of this vitamin. However, once fresh citrus fruits were added to their diets, scurvy ceased to be a problem.

Vitamin C is made from glucose, a simple sugar found in ordinary table sugar. In order to turn the glucose into vitamin C, a special liver enzyme is required. Humans do not have that enzyme in their systems, requiring them to take in vitamin C from an outside source, such as oranges. Most other animals do have the ability to convert sugar into this necessary vitamin.

Most of the research relating to vitamin C has dealt with the issue of whether or not it can cure or prevent the common cold. Since there are at least 113 distinct viruses known to be able to cause a cold, it is unlikely that any one vitamin could work to limit all the viruses. However, it does seem to have some positive effects in protecting against colds. This may be due to the effects of collagen building. Collagen is the substance essential to many body tissues including bone and blood vessel walls.

Excess vitamin C intake should be avoided by pregnant women, as it has been found that women who have taken a high dosage of this vitamin may give birth to children who have scurvy. The child's metabolism becomes adjusted to the excess, so the excess is then required in order for the child to remain normal. A Russian study, published in 1964, found that sixteen out of twenty pregnant women who took 6,000mg of vitamin C daily suffered abortions.

Another aspect of excessive vitamin C ingestion is its possible link with anaemia. A study by the National Institute of Arthritis, Metabolism and Digestive Diseases found that large amounts of vitamin C destroy the vitamin B12 contained in food. So a daily ingestion of half a gram or more of vitamin C may result in anaemia in some people.

One particular group of people may require more vitamin C than the rest of the population: smokers. This may not seem surprising in light of the earlier discussion of the protective effects of vitamin C as an antioxidant. It has been shown that smokers have lower blood levels of vitamin C than non-smokers,[14] and smokers with a vitamin C deficiency have a greater chance of developing certain oral mucosal lesions.[15]

Vitamin D

Vitamin D is seldom found to be deficient in the Western diet. However, toxic levels do occur. Vitamin D toxicity has been found in cases where the daily dose is 2,000 IU, five times the minimum requirement of 400 IU. The suggested maximum is 1,000 IU.

Among the dangers of excessive vitamin D in children are mental retardation and damage to internal organs. Since milk, margarine, butter and many breakfast cereals are high in vitamin D, parents should watch this intake closely. Being in the sun is another way to get your vitamin D. The ultraviolet rays of sunlight convert a substance under the skin into the vitamin. However, a lack of the vitamin in children can cause bone and teeth problems, as vitamin D is required to bind calcium to the bones and teeth. A lack of vitamin D in adults may cause depression.

Vitamin E

Vitamin E, like vitamin C, has many advocates who claim unproven benefits from its use. For example, vitamin E may be able to help cells live longer. This does not mean that vitamin E will slow the ageing process, but it may indicate that the vitamin, because of its antioxidant properties, can be a shield to certain environmental stresses, such as smog, radiation and other pollutants. When cells treated with vitamin E were exposed to these environmental stresses, only 30 per cent stopped reproducing compared to 90 per cent of the untreated cells. Other studies done at the University of Southern California have indicated that vitamin E may help to prevent emphysema and offer protection from smog by protecting both the lung tissue cells and the red blood cells as they pass through the lungs.

For over 25 years it has been recognized that the heart benefits from adequate amounts of vitamin E. There is also now evidence that it increases endurance (stamina) especially in those who are not well conditioned. It has also been found to reduce muscular injuries because of its antioxidant properties.

MINERALS

Minerals are usually structural components of the body, but they sometimes participate in certain body processes. The body uses many minerals – phosphorus, calcium and magnesium for strong teeth and bones; zinc for growth; chromium for carbohydrate metabolism; and copper and iron for haemoglobin production.

Iron

Iron is used primarily in developing haemoglobin, which carries the oxygen in the red blood cells. Women need more iron than men until they go through the menopause (18mg a day), at which time their iron requirements drop to that of men (10mg a day). Iron deficiency, common in women athletes, may impair athletic performance and should be corrected with supplementation.[16]

In the West, iron toxicity (an excess of iron) is rare, but the Bantu tribe of Africa experiences iron toxicity. This is because they cook in iron utensils and they brew their alcohol in iron, thereby greatly increasing their iron intake. There is some recent, yet still controversial, evidence that an excess of iron may increase the risk of heart disease.

Magnesium

Magnesium is the eighth most abundant element on the earth's surface and the fourth most abundant mineral in the body. It seems to help activate enzymes that are essential to energy transfer, so is important in strength and endurance activities. When it is not present in sufficient amounts, twitching, tremors and undue anxiety may develop. There is some evidence to indicate that people who are exercising should have an increased amount of magnesium.

Calcium

Calcium is primarily responsible for the building of strong bones and teeth. A diet that is chronically low in calcium therefore has a negative effect on bone strength, which leads to brittle and porous bones as one gets older, a condition known as osteoporosis. This condition is diagnosed when the bone density shows a loss of 40 per cent of the necessary calcium.

It occurs quite frequently in older people, especially post-menopausal women (including post-hysterectomy women), as oestrogen seems to serve a protective function against bone loss.[17] In addition, post-menopausal women exposed to excess thyroid hormone are at a greater risk of developing osteoporosis due to the increased loss of bone density seen in this population.[18] In fact, osteoporosis affects 25 per cent of women and 13 per cent of men over age 65.

The intake of adequate calcium (which may be higher than the current RDA) during the teenage and young adult years can aid in the development of peak bone mass, which may help to prevent osteoporosis later in life.[19] Another contributing factor to osteoporosis is the imbalance of phosphorus to calcium in the Western diet. Calcium and phosphorous work together, and should be consumed in a one to one ratio. However, the typical diet is much higher in phosphorus than calcium, leading to a leeching of calcium from the bones to make up for this imbalance.

Calcium is also necessary for strong teeth, nerve transmissions, blood clotting and muscle contractions. Without enough calcium, muscle cramps often result. It has been predicted that we will experience a great increase in gum disease in addition to weak bones because of our dietary increase in phosphorus over the last three to four decades.

Fluoride

Fluoride deficiency may be a primary nutritional deficiency in many parts of the Western world, resulting in cavities and dental caries. Fluoride helps to build stronger bones and teeth. The average citizen has 10.2 cavities. However, in Colorado Springs, where the water registers two parts per million of fluorides, the cavity rate is 0.61. In Newburgh, New York, dental caries rates were reduced by

60 per cent after adding one quart per million of fluoride to the drinking water.

Potassium

Potassium is a chief mineral in cell growth. A deficiency can cause impaired nerve and muscle functions ranging from paralysis to minor weakness, loss of appetite, nausea, depression, apathy, drowsiness, confusion, heart failure and even death.

Studies have shown an increase in blood pressure when sodium intake is high; such studies have also shown that blood pressure is decreased when the potassium intake is increased. A one to one ratio of sodium to potassium is considered good – although our foraging ancestors, who did not add table salt to their foods, may have been getting 10 times as much potassium as sodium. For most people, their sodium intake is much higher than desirable and their potassium intake too low.

Copper

Copper helps in the production of red blood cells. It also helps in the metabolism of glucose (sugar), with the release of energy, in the formation of fats in the nerve walls, and in the formation of connective tissues. Deficiency of copper is very rare.

Manganese

This mineral is used in fat and carbohydrate metabolism, pancreas development, prevention of bone defects, muscle contraction and many other functions. It has not yet been observed as a human deficiency.

Zinc

Zinc is an ingredient in insulin and is used in the carbohydrate metabolism that is necessary for energy. It also plays an essential part in protein metabolism, so is necessary for the normal growth of general organs, the prevention of anaemia and the growth of all tissues. It also helps in wound healing. It is seldom found to be deficient in diets in Western Europe or the US, but it has been observed to be deficient in some people in the Middle East. People on low-calorie diets may also be low in this mineral. However, zinc in excess of the RDA interferes with copper absorption and decreases the level of HDL ('good') cholesterol in the blood. The RDA for zinc is 12mg per day for women and 15mg for men.

Chromium

This essential mineral is necessary in small amounts to maintain normal blood sugar balance. Both men and women need about 120µm per day. If you have diabetes and are deficient in chromium, supplementation may help you control your blood sugar. Although chromium deficiency is not the primary cause of diabetes in the West, if you have a family history of mature-onset (Type II) diabetes, you should eat chromium-rich foods such as whole-grain breads, nuts, prunes, molasses, cheese and oysters, or consider taking a daily tablespoon of brewer's yeast.

Some people believe that chromium helps to build muscle and to burn fat, but there is no scientific evidence for either belief.

Selenium

Selenium is a powerful antioxidant that works with vitamin E. The RDA for selenium is 55µm for women and 70µm for men. It is unclear whether extra selenium is helpful in reducing the risk of cell damage among heavy exercisers. Because intakes greater than 200µm may be toxic, the best advice to date is to limit selenium intake to the RDA. Good food sources are meat, eggs, milk, seafood and – depending on the amount of selenium found in soil – broccoli, garlic, mushrooms and whole-grain cereals.

Trace Minerals

Trace minerals are those that are found in very small amounts. Nearly every element found in the body is 'essential', but the trace minerals are required in such small amounts that there is little reason for dietary deficiency. Usually foods high in calcium and iron contain the other necessary trace minerals.

Some athletes and heavy exercisers believe that they need high doses of minerals to counter the stress of hard training. However, most studies show that, except for iron (particularly among female athletes), the mineral status of highly trained athletes is similar to that of healthy, untrained people and that training does not deplete mineral status.

PHYTOCHEMICALS

Phyto- (Greek for 'plant') chemicals include thousands of chemical compounds which are found in plants. Some of these are vitamins and many have no known effect on us; however, more and more are being found to be highly beneficial.

In the past, the phytonutrients were classified as vitamins: flavonoids were known as vitamin P, cabbage factors (glucosinolates and indoles) were called vitamin U, and ubiquinone was vitamin Q. Tocopherol somehow stayed on the list as vitamin E. Vitamin designation was dropped for the other nutrients because specific deficiency symptoms could not be established – 'vita' means 'life' so if the compound could not be found to be absolutely essential for life it was no longer classified as a 'vitamin' but became a phytochemical.

Checklist for Foods with Anti-Cancer-Acting Phytochemicals

- *Highly effective:* garlic, carrots, celery, soya beans, cilantro, cabbage, parsley, ginger, parsnips, liquorice.
- *Moderately effective:* onions, flax, citrus fruits, broccoli, cauliflower, Brussels sprouts, tomatoes, peppers, brown rice, turmeric, whole wheat.
- *Somewhat effective:* oats, oregano, barley, basil, cantaloupe, berries, mint.

(Adapted from; Clark, K. 'Phytochemicals protect against cancer', *ACSM Health and Fitness Journal*, May/June 1998. p.35.)

Various phytochemicals have been found to reduce the chance of cancers developing, reduce the risk of heart attack, reduce blood pressure and increase immunity factors. Few of these have been produced in pill form, such as vitamin pills, so they must be consumed in fruits and vegetables daily. It is suggested that each of us consume at least five servings of raw fruits or vegetables daily. Since many of the phytochemicals are heat sensitive, cooking can destroy some or all of the active ingredients.

We are a long way from developing effective phytochemical supplements because there are so many elements which may be destroyed during processing. Garlic pills, for example, are available, but with deodorization some of the active ingredients have been removed – they were in the chemicals which gave the garlic its aroma.

Several types of phytochemicals are being studied (*see* box overleaf).

Recent research is confirming suspicions of the effects of soy products and related foods which have long been used in the Oriental diets. The observation that Oriental women did not experience the problems of menopause

Some Phytochemicals Currently under Study

Phytochemical	*Foodsource*
Polyphenols (flavonoids; e.g., quercetin)	Onions, garlic, red wine, tea (especially green)
Indoles	Cruciferous vegetables*
Isothiocyanates (e.g., sulforaphane)	Cruciferous vegetables, especially broccoli
Carotencios	Orange, yellow, and green vegetables; from fruits
Allyl sulphides	Onions, garlic, leeks, chives
Isoflavones (e.g., genistein)	Legumes (e.g., soyabeans)
Monoterpenes (e.g., limonene)	Oils from citrus fruits; nuts, seeds
Phytic acid	Whole grains, legumes
Lignan	Seeds; some fruits and vegetables
Ellagic acid	Grapes
Caffeic acid, ferulic acid	Fruits
p-Coumaric acid, chiorogenic acid	Fruits and vegetables
Glutathione	Fruits and vegetables (also freshly prepared meats)

* Cruciferous vegetables include broccoli, Brussels sprouts, cabbage, cauliflower, collards, kale, kohlrabi, mustard greens, rutabaga, turnip greens and turnips.

that Western women commonly endure, such as hot flushes, had long been known but no theories had yet been developed. Now we realize that a major factor is the fact that the Asians eat more vegetables, particularly soy beans.

It is the phytoestrogens, plant chemicals which mimic the effects of the female hormone oestrogen, which seems to be the major factor. These plant-like oestrogens have similar effects to the natural oestrogen in reducing heart disease, maintaining brain functions, reducing the incidence of breast cancers, and reducing the softening of the bones (osteoporosis). Additionally other positive effects, which may or may not be related to oestrogen intake, also occur, such as reductions in cancers (prostate, endometrial, bowel) and the effects of alcohol abuse.[20]

Plant Sterols

Plant sterols are somewhat similar to the animal sterol cholesterol but are unsaturated. These plant sterols compete for the same sites and thereby lower the blood cholesterol levels, often by 10 per cent. Soya is a good source for such sterols. Most green and yellow vegetables, and particularly their seeds, contain essential sterols.

Phenols

Phenols have the ability to block specific enzymes which cause inflammation. They also modify the prostaglandin pathways and thereby protect blood platelets from clumping thereby reducing the risk of blood clots. The blue, blue-red and violet colorations seen in berries, grapes and purple aubergine are due to their phenolic content.

Flavonoids

Flavonoids is the name for a large group of compounds. They are found primarily in tea, citrus fruits, onions, soya and wine. Some can be irritants, but others seem to reduce heart attack risk. For example, the phenolic substances in red wine inhibit oxidation of human LDL. The biological activities of flavonoids include action against allergies, inflammation, free radicals, liver toxins, blood clotting, ulcers, viruses and tumours.

Terpenes

Terpenes such as those found in green foods, soya products and grains, comprise one of the largest classes of phytonutrients. The most intensely studied terpenes are carotenoids – as evidenced by the many recent studies on beta carotene. Only a few of the carotenoids have the antioxidant properties of beta carotene. These substances are found in the bright yellow, orange and red plant pigments vegetables such as tomatoes, oranges and pink grapefruit contain.

Limonoids

These are a subclass of terpenes found in citrus fruit peels. They appear to protect lung tissue and aid in detoxifying harmful chemicals in the liver.

WATER

Water is called the essential non-nutrient because it brings with it no nutritional value and yet, without it, we would die. Water makes up approximately 60 per cent of the adult body, while an infant's body is nearly 80 per cent water. Water is used to cool the body through perspiration, to carry nutrients to the cells and waste products from them, to help cushion our vital organs, and is a constituent in the make-up of all body fluids.

The body has about 18 sq ft (1.6 sq m) of skin containing about two million sweat glands. On a comfortable day, a person will lose about half a pint of water in perspiration. Somebody exercising on a severely hot day may lose as much as 7 litres of water. This needs to be replaced or severe dehydration can result. It is therefore generally recommended that each person daily drink eight 8oz (500dl) glasses of water, or its equivalent, in other fluids. This amount is dependent upon the climate in which you live, the altitude at which you live, the type of foods that you eat, and the amount of activity that you participate in on a day-to-day basis.

CHAPTER 8
Applying Our Knowledge to the Dinner Table

Sensible eating requires an understanding of the basic principles of nutrition discussed in the previous chapters. The nutrients must appear in the diet in proper quantities, and the calories must be the amount necessary to maintain the proper weight. If proper weight is not maintained, then obesity may develop and diseases associated with obesity, such as diabetes, high blood pressure and heart disease, can begin.

There are other factors that the sensible eater must understand. Caloric needs change according to climate and the amount of activity in which the person participates. It is obvious that hot weather necessitates a greater intake of fluids due to the loss of water through perspiration. However, there is also a lesser need for calories, because the body does not need to burn as many calories to maintain its normal temperature.

A person using a great many calories, such as an athlete, needs more carbohydrates, but it is a myth that athletes need a great deal more

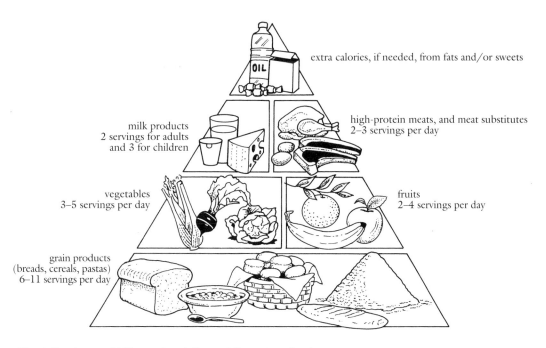

extra calories, if needed, from fats and/or sweets

milk products
2 servings for adults
and 3 for children

high-protein meats, and meat substitutes
2–3 servings per day

vegetables
3–5 servings per day

fruits
2–4 servings per day

grain products
(breads, cereals, pastas)
6–11 servings per day

Fig 6. Food pyramid illustrating daily need for various food groups.

protein than non-athletes. While the caloric needs may nearly double for the athlete who is expending a great deal of energy, the protein needs are increased only slightly, usually less than 30 per cent. Nor do people who exercise require more vitamins and minerals than others. Supplements given to athletes already consuming well-balanced diets have not been shown to improve performance.

Sensible eating also requires that we know how to prepare food, that we don't overspend our money on food, and that we are aware of the food fads that keep cropping up in our culture. We also need to give some thought to how we might effectively lose weight if we're overweight.

It is also important to know the effect of various foods on the teeth and on other organs, how we might prevent some of the food-borne diseases, and also how we might prevent diseases that may be caused by an improper diet.

EATING AND OVEREATING

Why do you eat? At least part of the answer lies in the feeding centre of the brain. When you begin to eat, the sugar content of the blood goes up, and the hypothalamus turns off. This part of hunger comes from your biological clock – you expect to eat at certain times of the day. If you go through the lunch hour without eating, you will be very hungry at the time, but as time passes, you will generally become less hungry. The hunger pangs that come from stomach contractions are learned and almost any habit that is learned can be unlearned if you go about it in the right way.

If you were to continue not eating, the experience of hunger would rise to a maximum in three to five days as the brain and muscles of the stomach continue to learn that food simply is not going to be coming along

as it once did. The stomach contractions will slow down and eventually cease almost entirely. Your body can be trained not to be hungry. The first three days of starvation or the first three days of a diet are the worst. It isn't that your stomach shrinks, but that you learn not to be hungry and your hypothalamus learns to adjust to lower blood sugar levels.

Most of us eat a little more than we need and the extra calories generally find their way to our hips. Some people are only somewhat overweight, some are obese. Obesity is often caused by overeating to an extreme degree. Commonly it is a result of an adjustment to stress. However, as we adjust to stress by eating, quite often we create more stress, because we are gaining weight. In many cases, we try to compensate for this stress by eating more because it may be food that we turn to as a solace to our stress.

Some people are obese because of physical problems, and there are medical procedures that can help them. In cases where the metabolism has slowed down, perhaps because of an underactive thyroid gland, doctors can administer the proper hormone to increase metabolism back to what is considered a 'normal' range.

Another problem can be the number of fat cells in a person's body. These are determined by both heredity and environment. The early years, even the early months, can be very important in determining the number of fat cells that a person will have.

Fat cells in an obese person may be three times as large as those in a lean person. Dieting may make the fat cells reduce in size, but not in number. The thinner cells just sit around waiting to be fed. Since it is the amount of fat that a person carries on his/her body that is the true culprit of disease, it is preferable to refer to being overfat as a health risk rather than being overweight. Many body builders may be overweight when compared to the height/weight charts commonly used to measure health risks by insurance companies, but they are not overfat.

There are many methods of determining if one is overfat. The most common method is to look at yourself in a mirror. If you look fat, you may be fat. Another way is to pinch the fat in certain areas of the body using skin callipers to assess how much fat you have overall. Without going to a professional, a quick assessment could be done by pinching the back of your upper arm to see if you have ⅜in (1cm) or more of fat. This could indicate that you are overfat. A ½in (1.3cm) of loose fat or loose skin at the waist could be another indication. Professionals usually will measure the amount of fat you carry in four to seven designated spots on the body (front and back of the upper arm, upper chest, upper back, stomach, hip and front of the thigh) and determine an overall percentage of body fat. Because men carry their fat predominantly in the stomach, while a woman's fat is distributed mostly in the thighs and buttock area, there are different sites of measurement for men and women.

Once your body fat percentage has been determined, you can then find out what a healthy weight would be for you. Men are usually considered healthy if their body fat is in the range of 10 to 15 per cent, while women are healthy if they fall between 20 to 25 per cent body fat. Women require more fat than men due to need of the menstrual cycle – if a woman falls below 12 per cent body fat, she will become amenorrhoeic (lose her regular menstrual cycle).

Of people who are overfat, one in twenty is so because of a physical malfunction, such as an underactive thyroid, a problem with the hypothalamus or in one of the other centres of the brain that deals with whether or not we feel full or hungry. But most of us are overfat because we eat too much. The need for food is innate. The urge to eat a certain kind of food, such roast beef or a milk shake, is a learned response. We learn our eating habits from our psychological conditionings. If our parents gave us compliments when we cleaned our plates when we were little, a pattern might have begun that made us believe that eating is good, and that we should eat everything on our plates even though we were actually satiated earlier. However, according to the Harvard University Nutrition Department, most people are overfat because they lack exercise, not because they overeat.

Those who are overfat can develop many problems such as osteoarthritis (from excessive wearing of the joints due to the continual carrying of the excess weight), diabetes mellitus (from excessive blood sugar), high blood pressure and hardening of the arteries. However, thinness is not the universal answer as some people function better when they are overweight.

Being overfat will probably speed up our death. There is evidence to indicate that fat people possibly 'live faster' than thin people. Studies with rats have found that the fat rat babies lived faster. Their sexual maturity was gained quicker, their running ability, their peak body weight and even death all occurred sooner than normal. Overfat people also tend to develop diabetes and kidney and heart problems earlier, and to have less resistance to infection.

THE DANGERS OF BEING OVERFAT

The Metropolitan Life Insurance Company has published the results of an extensive evaluation by the Society of Actuaries. Based on your weight as normally dressed and given your body frame, you should be in the appropriate weight range, or lower. Keep in mind, though, that this chart does not account for your body

fat; however, unless you are extremely muscled, these guidelines will give you an idea as to
how healthy your weight is for you.

Any weight over the ideal range increases
your chances of dying within your age group.
Obviously, few 18 year-olds die from diseases
caused by their obesity. However, many people over 40 die, and the proportion of deaths
increases each year. Therefore, the older a
person is, the greater are the chances of dying
because of being overweight. In using the
measures from the chart, if you are 15 to 24
per cent overweight, your chances of dying
are increased by 30 per cent over the normal
death rate for your age group. If you are 25 to
34 per cent overweight, your chances of dying

are increased by 45 per cent for your age
group. If you are over 35 per cent overweight,
your chances of dying are increased by 60 per
cent over your age group norm. If your
abdominal girth is two inches greater than
your expanded chest girth, you have a 'pot
belly' and your chances of dying are increased
an additional 50 per cent. If, for example, you
are 40 per cent overweight and have a 'pot
belly,' your chances of dying are increased
110 percent over the normal death rate for
your age group.

Another way to determine whether you are
overweight is to find your Body Mass Index.
On the chart draw a line between your height
and your weight to find your Body Mass Index.

Weights Based on Body Frame

Weights at ages 25 to 29 based on lowest mortality. Weights in pounds, shoes with 1-inch heels.

MEN Height Feet	Inches	Small frame	Medium Frame	Large Frame	WOMEN Height Feet	Inches	Small frame	Medium Frame	Large Frame
5	2	128–134	131–141	138–150	4	10	102–111	109–121	118–131
5	3	130–136	133–143	140–153	4	11	103–113	111–123	120–134
5	4	132–138	135–145	142–156	5	0	104–115	113–126	122–137
5	5	134–140	137–148	144–160	5	1	106–118	115–129	125–140
5	6	136–142	139–151	146–164	5	2	108–121	118–132	128–143
5	7	138–145	142–154	149–168	5	3	111–124	121–135	131–147
5	8	140–148	145–157	152–172	5	4	114–127	124–138	134–151
5	9	142–151	148–160	155–176	5	5	117–130	127–141	137–155
5	10	144–154	151–163	158–180	5	6	120–133	130–144	140–159
5	11	146–157	154–166	161–184	5	7	123–136	133–147	143–163
6	0	149–160	157–170	164–188	5	8	126–139	136–150	146–167
6	1	152–164	160–174	168–192	5	9	129–142	139–153	149–170
6	2	155–168	164–178	172–197	5	10	132–145	142–156	152–173
6	3	158–172	167–182	176–202	5	11	135–148	145–159	155–176
6	4	162–176	171–187	181–207	6	0	138–151	148–162	158–179

Source: Reprinted courtesy *Statistical Bulletin*, Metropolitan Life Insurance Company.

OBESITY AS A LIFE-THREATENING CONDITION

At the European College of Sports Medicine Convention in 1997 there was a major debate on whether obesity or a lack of physical fitness was the most negative risk factor in early death. Dr Claude Bouchard of Canada, one of the world's leading researchers on the effects of obesity, debated Dr Steven Blair of the United States, the world's leading researcher in the area of fitness. There is strong evidence that either obesity or lack of physical fitness is the number one cause of the diseases which leads to our deaths. Each agreed that obesity is often caused by inactivity. And each agreed that both are important factors in determining when and how one will die. An intelligent person will therefore do what is possible to reduce obesity while increasing physical activity.

At the World Congress of Sports Medicine in Orlando, Florida (1 June, 1998) Dr Bouchard presented some new evidence relative to weight gain and eating. While theoretically a person will gain 1lb (0.45kg) for every 3,500 calories he or she consumes over what it takes to live and move, studies have showed that with the same intake of calories (1,000 per day) over what was needed to keep the status quo, some people gained 9lb (4kg), while others gained over 26lb (13kg). Dr Bouchard's message is that heredity is very important in many aspects of our health. Still, the Lord does not help those who help themselves and help themselves and help themselves!

TO LOSE WEIGHT

Not everyone needs to diet, but if you wore all white to a party and the hostess showed home movies on you – it might be a hint! To lose weight, you might be able to change your eating habits by eating smaller and more frequent meals. There is evidence that eating four or five small meals a day is better than eating two or three large ones. Studies have been done with chickens and humans, and it has been found that nibblers, often called 'grazers', gain less weight than those who eat three times a day.

In order to lose 1lb (0.45kg) of fat per week, you must have a net deficit of 700 calories per day. This is because 1lb of fat contains 3,500 calories. You may choose to achieve this solely by decreasing your food intake by 700 calories per day. However, if this is your approach, be warned: your metabolism will slowly decrease over time to take into account the decrease in food energy, making it harder and harder for you to lose the fat. It would be much easier to lose weight if the replacement parts were not so readily available – in the pantry and refrigerator.

You may also choose to increase your activity level to burn off 700 calories a day. However, keep in mind that it takes a great deal of energy to achieve this goal, and it can be dangerous to embark on such a strenuous exercise programme if you are not currently exercising. Therefore, it is best to combine both to achieve your goal. Exercise will keep your metabolism up as you lose the fat, and you won't have to restrict your calories to such an extreme because you will be burning off energy each time you exercise. Examples of the number of calories you burn per pound per hour doing various activities are detailed in the box on p.70.

We now know that calories are used both during and after exercise. The longer and more vigorous the exercise, the longer one's basal metabolism is increased, and the more hours after you have exercised that you will continue to use more than the normal number of calories. A vigorous half an hour session of exercise, such as running or aerobic dance, can increase the number of calories used for

	Calories Burnt in Various Exercises	
	Calories per pound per hour	*Calories expended by a 150lb (68kg) person during 20 minutes of exercise*
Sleeping	0.36	18
Sitting at rest	0.55	27.5
Sitting at work	0.60	30
Light exercise		
Housework	1.0	50
Walking	1.2	60
Jogging	1.75	87.5

the next 4 to 6 hours. Some people think that exercising will make them eat more. This is not true. In fact, by exercising just before a meal, you can dull your appetite and decrease your desire for more calories.

Perhaps the most effective and practical manner of losing weight by dieting is through behaviour modification. This is a highly effective approach advocated by the behaviourist school of psychology. Several things can be done. First, the person has to become aware of how much food is being eaten, then the food can be eaten more slowly or in smaller portions. It takes about 20 minutes for the stomach to inform the brain that it has had enough food. If a person eats intelligently for the first 20 minutes of a meal, the time can be used to turn the brain off before a great deal of food has been consumed. A person may learn to savour the food differently, no longer gulping, but being conscious of the taste. Enjoy every bite, perhaps setting the fork down between bites. People can also learn to substitute food, such as a big salad and clear broth for filling sweets and fatty meats.

Before you can change your eating habits, however, you must be aware of exactly what you are doing. Behaviour modification experts generally suggest that you keep a dietary diary

for at least a week. Some experts suggest that it should be kept for as long as 5 months. Record everything you eat and drink and note exactly when and where you were when you were eating. You may find that you feel the urge to eat while you are studying, or when the television is on, or whenever you pass the refrigerator. Note what it was that you were thinking or feeling just before you began eating. Also note who was near you.

After you have completed your dietary diary, look for patterns in your behaviour. Do you like to eat in bed? Do you eat in your car, or while you are in the kitchen? If so, you may have to modify your behaviour to avoid eating in these places. You might make a rule that you will eat only while sitting at the dining room table with the television turned off. Or maybe your rule would be that you will snack only in the hall. The idea of this is to make you aware of the patterns you have established – so that you are conscious of when, where and why you are eating – and to change them.

You may change your eating times. Instead of breakfast at 7 o'clock, lunch at 12 and dinner at 6, you may try to fool your hypothalamus and stomach muscles. Let your stomach growl at 7, then eat something at 8 o'clock. Then you might try having a small lunch at

11:30. Your stomach muscles should be too embarrassed to growl at noon. You might sneak a snack at 5 o'clock and fool your hypothalamus again. Since we have been conditioned, like Pavlov's dogs, to eat at certain times, we often need to unlearn these habits.

Fat people tend to be more subject to external cues in their eating habits. In studies, when presented with a fear situation, fat people ate about the same amount of food that they would normally eat. Average-weight people ate less food. When told it was past their dinner time, fat people would eat more than normal; average-weight people would not eat unless they were hungry, or would eat very little. Average-weight people, when misled as to the time of day, would eat according to what their bodies told them, not according to what other people told them.

Fat people tend to be plate cleaners – they eat everything set before them whether or not they are hungry. If given small portions, the fat person will usually eat that and seldom ask for more. The average-weight people are much more likely to leave a little something on the plate.

You can use other psychological cues when dieting. You might put up a chart to list your daily food intake and exercise programme. You may also want to chart your weight every week. Remember, only *you* can be responsible for your weight loss, and it is up to you to take control of it. It is a good idea to set short- and long-term goals for yourself, and reward yourself every time you reach a goal. Keep in mind that hot fudge sundae may not be the best reward!

When dieting, it is generally wise to set small weight loss goals, rather then saying, 'I'm going to lose 70 pounds'. Set a goal of 3 to 5lb (1 to 2kg). When these goals are attained, give yourself a reward. This way, you'll achieve a frequent sense of success in your diet. A sensible diet requires a develop-ment of food habits that can be followed after the desired weight has been lost. A diet of 'rabbit food' and water is not going to be one you can stick to forever. It is important to remember that, even when dieting, you must give your body the nutrients that it needs.

Sensible dieting requires that you do not lose more than 2lb (1kg) a week. It is also necessary for you to develop food habits which can be followed after the desired weight loss. In developing an effective weight-loss programme, a person should make certain that there are sufficient amounts of high-quality protein, vitamins and minerals, and a minimum of fats and carbohydrates in the diet while reducing the number of calories.

Usually reducing some fat consumption (which saves 9 calories per gram), alcohol (which saves 7 calories per gram) and some carbohydrate consumption (which saves 4 calories per gram) will result in successful weight loss. Then combine this reduced calorie diet with both resistance training and aerobic exercise.

When you're dieting, have smaller portions of food and put them on a smaller plate, giving the visual effect of a full plate. Use a smaller glass for your skimmed milk, too. If you don't like leafy vegetables, a dieting staple, seduce your taste buds by flavouring them with various spices, but avoid butter. A Chinese cookbook may be helpful in this regard. And drink a lot of water.

Eliminate some foods at some meals. Instead of having potatoes every night, have them every other night. Make open-sandwiches instead of sandwiches using two slices of bread. (Some people use lettuce leaves instead of bread to make a sandwich.) Try substituting some foods for the high-fat foods – poultry, without the skin, for red meat and non-fat or low-fat frozen yogurt for ice cream.

It is too easy to add calories. A baked or boiled potato contains 100 calories. When mashed with milk, this goes up to 150 calories.

If butter and cream are added, the total goes up to 250, the same as French fries. Hash browns are 400 to 500 calories per serving because of the fat. Frying food can double the calories, depending on how much fat is absorbed. Broiling meats can reduce the calories because the fat drips out and is not eaten.

Reducing sweets, while it may not be palatable, is one of the most effective ways of limiting calories. For instance, use a sugar substitute to significantly reduce the number of calories consumed. You do not need to think of dieting as a system of starving yourself to death so that you can live longer. It really does not have to be self-punishment – be creative in your diet.

BEVERAGES

Beverages make up a large part of our diet. We often don't think too much about the types of liquids we drink. The most nutritious drinks have been rated by the US Center for Science in the Public Interest, which rated them according to the amount of fat and sugar, which would lower their rating, and the amount of protein, vitamin and mineral content, which would raise their rating. Their results were that skimmed or non-fat milk was rated a +47, whole milk +38 (the lower rating was because of its fat content), orange juice +33, Hi-C +4, coffee 0, coffee with cream –1, coffee with sugar –12, Kool-Aid –55, and soft drinks –92.

Milk

Milk is the best beverage for most people. Adults should drink two cups a day. Our need for milk can be satisfied by milk products, such as cottage cheese and yoghurt. Of course, the sugar and the cream in the ice cream give it a lower overall rating. In addition to its nutrient value as a developer of bones and organs, milk has been found to help people sleep. They go to sleep quicker, then sleep longer and sounder. Skim milk contains half of the calories of whole milk.

Coffee

Coffee contains several ingredients that may be harmful to the body. These include stimulants such as caffeine and the xanthines, oils which seem to stimulate the secretion of excess acid in the stomach, and diuretics that eliminate water from the body. Caffeine is found in coffee, tea and cola drinks. Brewed coffee contains 100 to 150mg of caffeine per cup, instant coffee about 90mg per cup, tea between 45 and 75mg per cup, decaffeinated coffee 2 to 4mg per cup, and cola drinks 40 to 60mg per cup. The therapeutic dose of caffeine given to people who have overdosed on barbiturates is 43mg. A one-half grain of Empirin contains 30mg yet a cup of coffee contains up to 150mg of caffeine.

Caffeine stimulates the central nervous system, and also elevates blood pressure and constricts the blood vessels. Both of these may assist in the development of high blood pressure. It has been reported that the caffeine in coffee, tea and cola drinks can produce the same symptoms as those found in a person who has reached a state of psychological anxiety. These symptoms include the following: nervousness, irritability, occasional muscle twitching, sensory disturbances, diarrhoea, insomnia, irregular heartbeat, a drop in blood pressure, and occasionally failures of the blood circulation system.

If someone has a heart problem, it may be wise to give up coffee. This is especially true if the person ingests five cups or more a day, since it can damage the central nervous system and elevate fatty acids and blood sugars in the blood, thereby burdening the blood vessels.

Coffee is an irritant. The oils in coffee irritate the lining of the stomach and the upper intestines. People who drink two or more cups of coffee per day increase their chances of getting ulcers by 72 per cent over non-coffee drinkers. Coffee, even with the caffeine removed, is no more soothing to the ulcer patient than the regular blend, because both types increase the acid secretions in the stomach. Since ulcer patients' acid secretion was not as high when caffeine alone was given to them as when they drank caffeine-free coffee, some other unknown ingredient in coffee may be responsible for increasing stomach acid levels.

Tea

Tea is not as irritating as coffee, but it does contain some caffeine and tannic acid, which can irritate the stomach. If you drink large amounts of tea, you should take it either with milk to neutralize the acid or add ice to dilute it.

Alcohol

There are 7 calories in a gram of alcohol. These calories contain no nutritional elements, but they do contribute to a person's total caloric intake. Since alcoholic drinks are surprisingly high in calories, they contribute greatly to the weight problems of many individuals. People who drink alcoholic beverages while eating a balanced diet will probably still consume too many calories. If they drink but cut down on eating, they may not develop a weight problem, but will develop nutritional deficiencies that can result in severe illness. Alcohol is also a central nervous system depressant, which causes a decrease in one's metabolism.

In addition to the normal dangers of alcohol, such as alcoholism and destruction of brain cells, there are other considerations. Beer or ale, because of their carbonation, have the effect of neutralizing stomach acid. This might increase the acids secreted by the stomach which could cause ulcers. Gin contains juniper berries and other substances that are stomach and intestinal irritants.

Studies have indicated that moderate alcohol consumption (less than three drinks a day) may increase the HDL type of blood cholesterol. While this may be true, one should consider that alcohol consumption is related to increased blood pressure and the additional calories may increase one's weight. Both of these are negatives in terms of heart disease.

The most effective alcoholic beverage for increasing the HDL cholesterols is cabernet sauvignan wine. The skins of the dark grapes add an extra antioxidant to the beverage. Of course, grape skins also contain such an antioxidant.

Beverages are Necessary for Rehydrating Your Body During and After Exercise

We all know that we must take in fluids during and after exercise. The question for many is 'Exactly what kind of fluid should I use?' A large number of studies have been done on this issue. It seems that carbohydrate (sugar such as glucose or maltodextrines, glucose polymers) and some electrolytes (sodium, potassium) are best. While the initial sweat contains sodium (salt), the amount of sodium in the sweat is reduced as the sweating continues, so high sodium content is not necessary in the fluid replacement drink, although some sodium is desirable.

The most effective drink contains both maltodextrines, as the sugar replacement, and some sodium and potassium. A 6 per cent level of sugars speeds water back to the muscles and other tissues. Look for a one-to-one relationship of sodium to potassium. The potassium helps to bring fluids to the tissues and to eliminate waste products from the muscles.

Some drinks will also add magnesium. This is very important. Like potassium, magnesium takes away the waste products from the muscles. However, it also helps to reduce cramping by relaxing the muscles. Make sure therefore that magnesium is in the drink, it should have about 300mg per serving.

Since alcohol is a diuretic it increases the amount of urine rather than keeping the fluid in the body where it is needed. It may taste good during or after a run, but it is counter-productive. Save your beer break until well after your practice or competition.

The body does not usually signal that it needs fluids until well after the need has existed. Most people will have some thirst after losing 1.5 to 2 per cent of their body weight in sweat – that is too late. We must take in fluids before, during and after a workout or a competition. Take in fluids at least every 15 minutes during practice or competition.

CHAPTER 9
Supplementing Your Diet

Contrary to some opinions, some pills may help you to live longer and better. Vitamin and mineral supplements are often helpful, especially those which include the antioxidants. Aspirin is also a major aid to health with only a few side-effects.

Too much of anything can cause problems. We need to look at the minimum amount of a substance which is needed, the ideal amount and the harmful amount. For example, the minimal amount of vitamin C required to prevent the bleeding disease 'scurvy' is 10mg a day. The minimum daily requirement generally listed as 30 to 50mg a day. If the antioxidant properties of vitamin C are important, even more of the vitamin may be desirable. Dr Ken Cooper, the man who coined the phrase 'aerobics' and began the fitness revolution in the 1960s recommends 1,000mg per day.[1] Some scientists have taken more than 2,000mg (2 g) a day without ill effects. However, some people have developed kidney stones from one of the binding elements used in making a vitamin C pill, although had they had enough water in their diet there would have been no problems.

Likewise, aspirin is useful in combating head and body pains and fever. It also is useful in reducing the pain of arthritis. But the major use of the drug today in the United States is in reducing the chances of a heart attack occurring by making the blood platelets more slippery so that they do not clump together and become blood clots. However, some people develop gastric bleeding from taking aspirin. About 4 per cent of people are susceptible to this problem. Statistics in the United States indicate that about 17,000 people die each year from the gastric bleeding caused by aspirin and other non-steroidal anti-inflammatory drugs such as ibuprofen (Advil), acetaminophen (Tylenol), and other such compounds. However, on the 'plus' side it appears that aspirin reduces the chances of developing cancer of the lower intestine or colon, and it may slow the onset of Alzheimer's disease.

For vitamin C and aspirin, the pluses definitely outnumber the minuses. But how does your body tolerate such chemicals? This is the key factor. If your mother died from gastric bleeding due to taking an aspirin-like compound and your father died of a heart attack, what are your odds in taking aspirin? You will undoubtedly want some medical tests to determine your susceptibility.

ASPIRIN AND OTHER NON-STEROIDAL ANTI-INFLAMMATORY DRUGS (NSAID)

Drugs such as aspirin, ibuprofen, indomethacin, naproxen and piroxicam are common types of anti-inflammatory drugs. They seem to have other functions as well.[2] Chronic inflammation has a key role in the abnormal processes related to ageing, including changes in body composition, congestive heart failure and possibly dementia. But aspirin also has properties which reduce the clotting abilities of the blood platelets, thereby reducing the risk of heart attack and strokes caused by clots. (However, it can increase the incidence of strokes whose cause is haemorrhage.) Recent evidence suggests that both heart attacks and strokes can be caused when the blood vessels are inflamed. Obviously these anti-inflammatory drugs can counteract such inflammation.

The six billion people in the world consume fifty billion doses of aspirin. Some, of course, are not eating their share! In the USA, aspirin is taken primarily to ward off heart attack. Nearly 38 per cent of aspirin doses are taken for this purpose. The recommended dose varies from half to one per day. Some people take an infant formula aspirin every day, some take a full aspirin every other day. Two major international studies have found that the risk of stroke is reduced by about 10 per cent with the use of aspirin.

Reducing arthritis pain is the second most common use of the drug. A little over 23 per cent of users take the drug for this reason. One famous physician with unbearable arthritis pain consumed a small bottle of aspirin daily to control his pain.

Controlling headache is the reason for another 14 per cent of the population taking the drug. The remainder of users take it to reduce fever or to control pains in other parts of their bodies.

Some, but not all, studies indicate that aspirin may help to ward off the dementia which is often associated with old age. Long-term use seems to improve mental functioning and ward off Alzheimer's disease.

A reduced breast cancer risk has been shown in some large studies, although not all studies have found the same risk reduction. And some studies find that aspirin may increase the risk of colorectal cancer, but, again, not all studies have found this. Since these drugs are known to be stomach and intestinal irritants it may be this negative quality which is responsible for irritations of the intestines and the possibility of developing a colorectal cancer. Of the NSAID-type drugs, low-dose ibuprofen is least likely to cause gastrointestinal complications. Buffered aspirin does not seem to have this same protective ability.

GINKGO BILOBA

Ginkgo biloba is one of the more ancient plants still living today. Extracts from its leaves were already used in ancient China, whereas in the Western world they have been utilized only since the 1960s when it became technically possible to isolate the essential substances of *Ginkgo biloba*. Pharmacologically, there are two groups of substances which are of some significance: the flavonoids, effective as free oxygen radical scavengers, and the terpenes (the ginkgolides) with their highly specific action in slowing blood clot formation.[3]

Ginkgo biloba seems to have the effect of stabilizing or reducing (in 20 per cent of cases) the effects of dementia which often comes with old age.[4]

Among the reasons given for its potential effectiveness are that it may:

- protect against brain cell damage by a chemical called glutamate which might allow excess calcium infiltration into brain cells;
- prevent a constriction of the brain's blood vessels;
- aid in keeping the blood vessels elastic.

In one study of people taking *Ginkgo biloba*, two out of three improved in their tests measuring attention, memory, behaviour and their abilities to perform the necessary activities of daily life. It seems to work not only in slowing or stopping brain deterioration but in preventing it.

THE ANTIOXIDANT SUPPLEMENTS

Beta Carotene

Beta carotene is a precursor to vitamin A. If you have not taken in sufficient vitamin A through milk, eggs, liver, cheese, butter or fish oil, six units of beta carotene can be converted into one unit of vitamin A. What is left acts as a strong antioxidant. It can lower the risk of cataracts – a clouding in the lens of the eye which blurs vision and often occurs with age. It also reduces the risk of many cancers,

particularly lung, bladder, rectal and the serious skin cancer called melanoma.

There is no recommended minimum daily requirement for this substance but the vitamin A which it can make has a minimum recommended daily amount of 4,000 IU for women and 5,000 for men. Dr Cooper's recommendation is 25,000 international units per day of beta carotene.[5]

Vitamin C

Vitamin C has a minimum daily requirement (MDR) or 'daily values' (DV) of 30 to 50mg. (60mg for smokers). It may make the cholesterol level more favourable by lowering total cholesterol while raising the good HDL. It is an antioxidant which may reduce the risk of

---

Antioxidant Supplementation

The Alliance for Aging Research (AAR), based on 200 clinical studies, recommends that people at high risk of cancer, especially asbestos workers and smokers, should not take any beta carotene supplements. For others interested in health promotion and disease prevention, they recommend the following ranges of supplements (in an ageing population): vitamin C, 250 to 1,000mg daily; vitamin E, 100 to 400 IUs daily; beta carotene, 17,000 to 50,000 IUs (10 to 30mg) daily.

The *University of California Wellness Letter*, based on the National Cancer Institute's findings, has withdrawn its recommendation for smokers to take beta carotene supplements, although they see no harm or benefit in non-smokers taking low doses if it's not obtained in the diet. Their recommendation: in addition to eating five or more servings of fruits and vegetables daily, take 200 to 800 IUs (133 to 533mg) of vitamin E daily; 250 to 500mg of vitamin C, but no more than 6 to 16mg of beta carotene daily for non-smokers not obtaining adequate amounts in their diet.

Dr Dean Ornish's Preventive Medicine Research Institute (PMRI) conducts pioneering research on lifestyle (diet, exercise, stress management and group support) and heart disease. Says PMRI's research director, Larry Scherwitz, PhD, 'if a three-day nutritional analysis reveals program participants are not obtaining adequate antioxidant levels in the diet, we recommend a range of supplementation: 1–3g vitamin C; 100 to 400 IUs of dry vitamin E daily; 10,000 to 25,000 IUs of beta carotene.'

The Kenneth Cooper Aerobics Center also espouses antioxidant supplementation – as an adjunct to consuming five or more servings of fruits and vegetables daily. The recommended amounts from food sources and supplements are. 1,000mg vitamin C, 15mg (25,000 IUs) beta carotene, and 400 IUs vitamin E (specifically d-alpha tocopherol – the natural form of vitamin E). Endurance athletes benefit from higher doses of antioxidants, and so the Center suggests that anyone exercising more than 5 hours weekly should double the recommended dosage to combat excess free radical by-products.)

---

cataracts. Some cancer risk may also be lessened (larynx, oesophagus, mouth, pancreas and stomach). In addition, by increasing immunity, it may reduce your chances of contracting infections such as a cold.

Many people have been taking 250 to 500mg daily for years, but Dr Cooper is now recommending 1,000mg per day as a supplement.[6] You can also get that amount by eating thirteen to seventeen oranges or forty-four tomatoes a day. Fifteen oranges will add 1,100 calories to your diet while the tomatoes will add 950, so if calories are a concern, the vitamin pill may be your better solution.

Vitamin E

Vitamin E is a strong antioxidant which also acts as an anticoagulant – that is, it reduces the blood's ability to clot, thereby reducing the risk of a coronary thrombus, a primary cause of heart attack, and brain embolisms, a primary cause of strokes. As with the other antioxidants, it reduces the risk of some cancers, of cataracts and it increases immunity to other diseases. In those who exercise, vitamin E also seems to reduce injuries to the small muscle fibres and may be important in preventing such conditions as 'shin splints'.

Reports in the *British Medical Journal*[7] indicate that 2,000 units of vitamin E delayed both the onset of Alzheimer's and the time of death. In the Cambridge Heart Antioxidant Study, 400 to 800 units of vitamin E daily considerably reduced the death rate from heart disease.

Vitamin E is measured in either international units (solid form foods) or milligrams (if in oils). They are roughly equivalent measures. While the minimum daily requirement is only ten IU's, Dr Cooper recommends 400 units per day,[8] and many people have taken more than double that without any apparent risk. If you want to take your 400 IU in foods you can eat 300 cups of instant oat cereal (43,500 calories), 6½lb (3kg) of potato chips (16,000 calories), or 32lb (14kg) of canned tuna in oil (31,000 calories). Since 3,500 calories will put on 1lb (0.45kg) of body weight for the average person, you will gain between 5 and 10lb (2.3 to 4.5kg) a day if you want to get 400 units of vitamin E through 'natural' sources. And the 'chemical' in the pill is the same chemical as is found in the oats or the tuna.

A recent study indicates another aspect of this desirable type of supplementation. Mortality from coronary heart disease in 50 to 54-year-old men was found to be four times higher in Lithuania than in Sweden. Most risk factors were similar between the men in the two countries. The major difference seemed to be in the antioxidant intakes, particularly vitamin E – the Lithuanians, intake was much lower. This corresponds with a study in England which showed that vitamin E supplements from 400 to 800 IU daily reduced the death rate from heart attacks by 47 per cent.[9]

Coenzyme Q 10

Coenzyme Q 10 (ubiquinone) is another antioxidant. It has been linked to DNA-related problems in both the nerves and the muscles.[10] It also works with both vitamin C and vitamin E in a number of actions in which all three are utilized together.[11]

As often happens, the research done by local scientists can influence the acceptance of the substance. While Q 10 has been studied in the United States, Dr Cooper does not recommend it as a daily antioxidant. On the other hand, the work of Jan Karlsson and others in Sweden makes Q 10 a favourite among the Nordic peoples. The Swedish National Food Administration recommends 2 to 20mg per day. Jan Karlsson recommends 50 to 100mg per day with élite athletes taking in 100 to 300mg per day.[12]

Selenium

Selenium is a mineral which is part of an essential enzyme (glutathione peroxidase) which protects a naturally occurring antioxidant (glutathione). It works with vitamins C, E and beta carotene. It may, as Vitamin E, reduce micro-injuries to the small muscle fibres. It may also reduce the risk of digestive cancers, especially of the stomach and oesophagus. In fact, it seems to be protective against all cancers. It is found in greater abundance in North American soils than in European soils. It therefore is found more often in both plants and animals raised in America.[13]

Side-effects of an excess of selenium can include hair loss, digestive problems (vomiting, diarrhoea, nausea), irritability, nerve cell problems and fatigue. Dr Cooper considers supplementation of selenium optional as long as you are getting 50 to 100mg a day. Natural sources include: 3.5oz (100g) of tuna (115mg of selenium); 0.5oz (14g) of tortilla chips (120mg of selenium); 3.5oz (100g) of lasagna noodles (96mg) or spaghetti (65mg). So it is quite easy to get this mineral in a normal diet. However, fruits and vegetables are quite low in selenium, while meats, grains and beans are generally high.

DESIRABLE ESSENTIAL FATTY ACIDS

The benefits of fish oils in reducing heart disease are common knowledge. These essential fatty acids (EFA) were given the name of 'vitamin F' in the 1920s. While desirable, they are no longer viewed as vitamins. These oils are part of the polyunsaturated fats (PUFA) group. Most people obtain enough of these fatty acids in their diets – particularly if they consume vegetable oils, meats, fish or poultry.

The most important of these EFAs are: linoleic, linolinic and arachidonic acids. Some vegetable oils contain linolenic acid but not eicosapentaenoic acid (EPA) or docosahexaenoix acid (DHA) which fish provide. Fish are able to convert linolenic acid into EPA and DHA. The human body does not have this ability. These fatty acids are precursors to the development of hormone-like substances called prostaglandins.

The one hundred prostaglandins have a number of functions. Some constrict or dilate the blood vessels (altering blood pressure), some affect the passages of messages along the nerves, some affect the excretion of water from the kidneys. One, called thromboxane, made from the fatty acid arachidonic acid, increases blood clotting. The EPA and DHA may also be implicated in the reduction of cholesterol and triglycerides (*see* Chapter 7), which reduce the risk of heart attack.

When your skin is cut you want your blood to clot quickly. However, clots in the blood are the major causes of heart attacks and cerebral vascular accidents. Clots are continually being made in the blood and are generally dissolved. However, if one sticks in an artery where it has been formed it is called a thrombus. If it is formed in the blood and floats to another area it is called an embolism. Most heart attacks are caused by a thrombus sticking in a coronary artery that nourishes the heart muscle. This is called a coronary thrombosis. Embolisms are often the cause of strokes as they float to an artery of the brain and cut off its blood supply, thereby deadening that area of the brain.

Years of observation and study have shown that people who eat lots of fish have fewer blood-clotting problems, and so fewer heart attacks and strokes. This is because the fatty acids in the fish fat change the production of thromboxane and thereby reduce the clotting ability of the blood.

Omega 3 Fatty Acids

There are actually six different omega 3 fatty acids, the most important of which are (alpha) linolenic acid, DHA and EPA. People who exercise heavily generally have lower than normal levels of omega 3 fatty acids, so it seems important for them, as well as for non-exercising people, to get plenty of this substance.

There are fish oil pills which can be consumed, but these do not seem to be as effective as actually eating fish. Also, the proper dosage of pills is not known and whether there are any adverse side-effects from their use. So here is one area where the 'natural' food seems better than the pill. You should consume fish about three times a week or more. It is also not known whether the benefits from eating fish derive only from the oil, or whether there is some hidden benefit from the non-oily parts of the fish. Still, fish oil supplements, from fish muscle, have been tried in a number of studies and have proved somewhat effective in reducing pain. The ideal dose seems to be 2 to 3g of omega 3 oil daily.[14]

It must be mentioned, however, that increasing the amount of omega 3 fatty acids requires a greater intake of vitamin E, because vitamin E is reduced when omega 3s are increased. Since the omega 3 fatty acids are more easily destroyed by oxidation, the antioxidant vitamins (E, C and beta carotene) are essential to protect them from disintegrating. The increase of omega 3 oils and antioxidants can reduce the less desirable omega 6 oils mentioned below. They can therefore reduce pain.

Omega 6 Fatty Acids

There are six omega 6 fatty acids, the most important of which are linoleic acid, arachidonic acid and the linolinic acid. This type of fatty acid appears to produce more of the inflammatory prostanoid types of by-products. In our Western diets, we seem to have much more of this fat than we need, and heavily exercising people in particular have more than normal in their blood. Present-day ratios range from ten to fifty times more of omega 6 than omega 3. The ideal range is under five to one[15] while our Stone Age ancestors were closer to a one to one ratio.

The higher rate of inflammatory products produced by too high a level of omega 6 fatty acids may be implicated in arthritis and other inflammatory diseases – such as those pains felt when exercising. We therefore don't need any more of this fatty acid. While we need some, we may get too much.

Calcium Supplementation

Calcitonin, a nasal spray, has been found to be effective in replacing lost calcium in the bones. This is particularly true for the lumbar spine area.[16]

BEING A WISE CONSUMER

A number of useless products are advertised in the media. For many, there is absolutely no scientific proof of their working – except for a possible placebo effect in which a person attains some benefits because he or she 'thinks' the product will help them.

For example, melatonin, which is prohibited in the UK but is still available in the US, has been touted as a substance which can 'strengthen the body's immune system' and is used to reduce the effects of jetlag. Many people take it daily, but the British Olympic Association does not recommend it.[17]

Shark cartilage is advertised as a substance which can inhibit the growth of cancer tumours. Various herbal concoctions have also been advertised as cures for a number of maladies and as substances which can make you feel better. Thousands of other types of 'alternative medicines' are advertised in the media and on the Internet.

DHEA (dehydroepiandrosterone) is not approved by the British National Formulary nor by the US Food and Drug Administration. It has been advertised as a hormone, a

---

Supplements

Buying supplements can be inexpensive or very expensive. In some countries they can only be purchased at pharmacies, while in others, the supermarkets carry some supplements which are less expensive. Health food stores generally carry supplements up to the dosage allowed by that country.

The United States generally allows higher levels of supplements than other countries. And with the American penchant for discounting, there are several mail order houses which are quite cheap. However, buying from outside of your country can create problems. For example, in Norway for high-dose vitamins you need a Norwegian doctor's prescription and a letter from a pharmacy that they do not carry such high doses.

Supplementing Your Nutritional Needs Through Vitamin or Mineral Pills
Buying vitamin pills should be determined by what you need. Some people need more of a vitamin than do others. For instance, if you were thinking of conceiving a child you might take some special vitamins, such as folic acid, which might decrease the chances of neural-tube defects in the baby. Some people may require a special kind of vitamin, such as a water-soluble vitamin A, for example. When restricting caloric intake for weight loss, it is a good idea to take a multivitamin and mineral supplement as it can be difficult to get all the vitamins and minerals you need while on a 'diet.'

Labelling is often confusing. Does the label state 100mg of magnesium gluconate or does it say 5.4mg of magnesium? Both mean the same in terms of meeting your body's requirements for magnesium. Does it state 325mg of calcium lactate or 42mg of calcium? Again, they both mean the same to your body.

When you purchase supplements, try to match the voids in your diet to the vitamin pill. You might have a knowledgeable doctor or a registered dietician analyse your diet, then get the exact dietary supplement or supplements that you need. Most people get sufficient amounts of vitamin D without a supplement but are often very low in magnesium, and most pre-menopausal women are low in iron, so you may want to include these in your supplement if you find that you are deficient in these. If you don't eat citrus fruits or tomatoes, you may be low in vitamin C. If you don't eat meat or wheat, you may be low in the B vitamins. And if you don't eat whole-grain cereals, you may be low in vitamin E.

Some vitamins, such as A, B1 and C, are inexpensive to produce in the amounts needed for our daily minimal requirements. Others, such as pyridoxine, niacin, pantothenic acid or vitamin E, are expensive; consequently, many inexpensive vitamin preparations have the inexpensive vitamins without having the other vitamins. Again, be sure you know what vitamins/minerals you need and in what doses, and then check to be sure that the supplement you have chosen best suits your needs.

---

sex stimulant and a life extender with a number of positive side-effects. Dr Mike Cullum, clinical director for oncology services at University Hospital, Birmingham, describes such claims as simply 'garbage'.

In a recent survey, 40 per cent of British consumers believed that many dietary supplements are actually medicines – even though the labels on the products may carry a disclaimer. Most of us need some supplementation of our diets, but as noted in Chapter 7, the phytochemicals are not yet found in many supplements. We must therefore be certain to eat at least five servings of fruits and vegetables daily. Those five servings will go a long way in providing you with your quota of beta carotene and vitamin C.

CHAPTER 10

Tobacco

R.J. Reynolds III, grandson of the founder of a tobacco company, died in 1994 from two diseases of smoking, emphysema and heart disease. Because of his health problems he had given up smoking in 1988, but it was too late. He was the fifth member of his family to die from smoking-related causes. His half brother Patrick conducted a memorial service in Los Angeles. Patrick had long ago sold all of his stocks in the tobacco company and had spent over $2.5 million of his inheritance in anti-smoking causes.[1]

Cigarette smoking is without a doubt the greatest single public health problem the West has ever faced. In 1964, the Surgeon General of the United States reported to the nation that cigarettes were definitely causative of lung cancer and many other lung diseases. That slowed up a few smokers, but the health risks of smoking keep mounting. A British study examining many of the causes of death found that the lowest risk was among those who had never smoked and those who had given up smoking.[2]

Tobacco use, not heart disease or cancer, is the number one killer of people in the United States.[3] This study looked at the environmental causes of death rather than the actual disease from which the person died. Tobacco use was found to cause 400,000 deaths for the year of 1990. Poor diet and lack of exercise together accounted for 300,000 deaths. The diseases which actually caused the physical death were: heart disease, cancers, strokes and low birth weights of the babies of smoking mothers. Together these accounted for 19 per cent of all deaths in the United States.

THE INGREDIENTS OF CIGARETTE SMOKE

In every 'balanced blend of fine aromas' in cigarette smoke, there are more than 4,000 different chemicals, forty of which have been proven to be carcinogenic.[4] Among these are acids, aldehydes, ketones, hydrocarbons, arsenic, carbon monoxide, nitrogen dioxide, nicotine, cancer-producing agents, ammonia, nitric oxide, benzene, hydrocyanic acid and tars. Tars carry these cancer-producing agents. The one-pack-a-day smoker inhales about 8oz (227g) (a half a pint of tar solids) into the lungs each year. At least 60 per cent of the material which is inhaled in every puff of smoke is therefore relatively deadly.

There is some evidence that smoking low-tar, low-nicotine cigarettes can reduce the amount of tar in the lungs. An American Cancer Society report showed that deaths from lung cancer were 26 per cent less among the low-tar cigarette smokers than among the high-tar cigarette smokers. Death from heart disease was 14 per cent less for the low-tar smokers. Other findings were that deaths from lung cancer for non-smokers were only 15 per cent of that for low-tar smokers. So low-tar smokers die from lung cancer about seven times more often than the non-smokers.

Nicotine

Nicotine is a fast-acting poison which is sometimes used in insecticides. Its effects on the body include: the mobilizing of fatty acids, which increases the cholesterol level of the blood; the constricting of blood vessels in the skin, which increases blood pressure; and the stimulation, then the depression, of the nervous system. As is now known, nicotine is highly addictive – second only to cocaine and its derivatives.

The lethal adult dose is 60mg. Depending on the brand, a cigarette contains 0.05 to 2.5mg, averaging under 1 per cent, of which 80 to 90 per cent reaches the bloodstream. A cigar contains 120mg (double the lethal dose), but a non-inhaling cigar smoker takes in only 20 to 50 per cent of the available nicotine.[5] Tobacco companies have been able to raise a type of tobacco which has a nicotine level of 6 per cent. It is illegal to grow this in the United States.[6]

Nicotine is metabolized in the liver. The metabolism takes about 25 minutes to break down half of the nicotine present. (This is called a half-life.) By the time the nicotine has been reduced to 30 to 50 per cent of the original dosage, the addicted smoker needs another dose.

Arsenic

This is a lethal poison. It has been greatly reduced in cigarettes during the last 15 years, yet the average smoker takes 40 to 50mg per day; 20 per cent of this is still present in the body after four days. It has an accumulative build-up, and arsenic in smoke has produced cancer in mice.

Benzene

Benzene is a highly toxic substance. In 1990 the Food and Drug Administration forced a recall of a famous mineral water because it was contaminated with benzene. A cigarette has about 2,000 times more benzene in it than did a bottle of that water. The use of benzene is also prohibited in the manufacture of several compounds, including paint thinner.

Benzopyrine

This is a carcinogenic agent found in both tobacco and marijuana. Its exact role in the human cancer process is not yet known, but studies of mice have shown cancer in both the adults and the babies of mice who were exposed to the substance.

Nitrogen Dioxide

Nitrogen dioxide (NO_2) is considered hazardous in air pollution when it reaches five parts per million. In cigarette smoke, it is 250 parts per million.

Carbon Monoxide

Exposure to 120 parts per million of carbon monoxide for one hour can cause dizziness, headache and exhaustion. Cigarette smoke contains 42,000 parts per million. Carbon monoxide poisoning (high carbo-oxi-haemoglobin) can also cause nausea and a lack of muscular coordination.

Hydrogen Cyanide

This works against respiratory enzymes. Long-term exposure above 10 parts per million is dangerous. Cigarette smoke contains 1,600 parts per million.

Ammonia

This substance is added to cigarettes to preserve and maintain the nicotine level.

IMMEDIATE EFFECTS OF SMOKING ON THE BODY

As soon as one takes a few puffs from a cigarette, the central nervous system is stimulated by nicotine. Nicotine first acts as a stimulant, then after it wears off the effect on the body is that of a depressant. This increases the need for another cigarette to restimulate the body. At the same time, nicotine acts like the neurotransmitter acetylcholine in the synapse of the nerves. This gives a calming effect. So cigarettes create both an 'upper' and a 'downer' effect at the same time. Nicotine is the only drug that gives two such strong actions simultaneously. This is why the withdrawal from it is so difficult. The addicted person withdraws with an upper reaction, as in a heroin withdrawal, from the depressant effects of not having the drug. Simultaneously, there is a crashing reaction, somewhat similar to that from cocaine, from the stimulant effects of the drug. While neither reaction is as strong as a withdrawal from heroin or cocaine, the combination withdrawal makes it very difficult to overcome. This is why nicotine is considered to be the third most difficult drug from which to withdraw – after crack cocaine and regular cocaine.

As noted, nicotine, which is found exclusively in tobacco, increases the adrenalin and adrenalin-like substances, which in turn increase blood pressure. This can be dangerous to anybody who has a tendency towards stroke or heart disease. The heart rate can be speeded up by as much as twenty beats per minute, thereby increasing the need for oxygen in the heart. However, because of the increased carbon monoxide in the blood, there is not sufficient oxygen for the heart's increased needs. This is believed to be a factor in the increased number of heart attacks among smokers. Nicotine also releases fats into the blood, especially cholesterol, so that the cholesterol level of the blood is raised. This increases the hardening of the arteries.

Hunger and the desire for food are generally reduced. Nicotine raises the blood sugar level, one of the things that gives people the feeling of energy. It also inhibits stomach contractions. In addition, it numbs the taste buds, so food doesn't taste as good.

It also shortens the blood-clotting time. In fact, one cigarette can hasten the blood-clotting time by as much as 25 per cent. This effect lasts from 15 minutes to 3 hours and is probably a prime reason for the increased heart attack rate in smokers. There is also a constriction of the arteries of the heart so that a smaller blood clot can block the blood flow.

Additionally, there is an effect on the respiratory system. Smoking constricts the bronchial tubes, which reduces the amount of air that can reach the lungs. Just one cigarette damages the lungs. It paralyses the cilia (hair-like organs) which carry dirt and other foreign substances from the lungs back to the nose and the mouth. In heavy smokers, the cilia have entirely disappeared.

The smoker's cough in the morning is due to the fact that the small hairs in the breathing passages, which have been anaesthetized by the smoke, have begun to come alive again. Their movements and the increased mucus, which is also developed by the smoking, tickles and irritates the breathing passages and causes the smoker to cough. This increase in mucus becomes a breeding ground for germs, possibly accounting for the increased number of colds in smokers.

Smoking also narrows the visual field and impairs a person's ability to drive at night. It also decreases athletic performance, especially in the endurance sports which require great stamina such as swimming, distance running, football and basketball.

Carbon monoxide is a very dangerous element in cigarette smoke. It combines with the haemoglobin, the iron compound in the red blood cells which transports the oxygen from the lungs to the cells. But since the haemoglobin has 200 times more affinity for the carbon monoxide than it does for oxygen, the carbon monoxide can starve out the oxygen, which is necessary to live. Carbon monoxide then becomes a poison because the oxygen in the carbon monoxide cannot be released to the cells. This makes the blood less efficient. As much as 10 per cent of a smoker's red blood cells can be made useless because they are carrying carbon monoxide rather than oxygen.[7] Any increase in carbon monoxide makes the heart pump faster, since more blood is needed to bring the necessary oxygen to the tissues. Carbon monoxide in cigarettes is 640 times greater than the level considered safe for industrial plants.

People who commit suicide by locking themselves in a garage and turning on the car engine die because the carbon monoxide in the car exhaust starves out the oxygen in the blood. When an excess of the gas is absorbed into the blood, a coma begins – and death will follow shortly as the percentage of carbon monoxide increases in the blood and starves the body's organs of the necessary oxygen.

The carbon monoxide in cigarette smoke can impair eyesight, manual dexterity, reflexes and the ability to estimate time intervals. These effects are worsened at higher altitudes. Because of the effects of carbon monoxide, the average smoker at sea level gets about the same efficiency from his lungs as does a non-smoker living at an altitude of 8,000ft (2,440m) above sea level.

A study done by the Environmental Protection Agency covering 29,000 people in 18 metropolitan areas showed the effects of pollution and smoking on the carbon-monoxide level of the blood. Suburban non-smokers showed from 0.4 to 1.5 per cent carbon monoxide in the blood. City-living non-smokers ranged from 0.8 to 3.2, averaging 1.5 per cent in their blood. Most of the non-smokers in Los Angeles, Denver, Chicago and San Francisco exceeded that 1.5 per cent average of carbon monoxide in the blood. If these people smoked, it added another 4 per cent to the carbon monoxide level, so Los Angeles smokers averaged 6.2 per cent carbon-monoxide, and some people measured over 10 per cent of blood carbon monoxide. Smokers with serious cardiovascular problems have their powers considerably impaired when their carbon monoxide level is over 3.5 per cent.

As a result of the reduced oxygen in the blood, smoking even one cigarette interrupts the body's production of collagen for 30 to 40 minutes. Collagen is a substance employed by the body to mend broken bones and other wounds, so smoking therefore slows the healing process. Collagen breakdown also causes wrinkles in the skin.

Smoking also reduces fertility in men and may increase impotency (inability to achieve an erection). Both occur because of low oxygen in the blood and a reduction of male hormones. Both are quickly reversible after stopping smoking. Female hormones are also reduced. This can cause menstrual irregularities, infertility and the growth of facial hair.

THE LONG-TERM EFFECTS OF SMOKING

Smoking increases the death rate to a great degree: it hardens the arteries; doubles the heart attack rate; increases the emphysema rate by four to six times; and increases the lung cancer rate by eight or more times. It also increases the chances of many other diseases. Smokers arrive at old age with 20 to 30 per cent less bone density than non-smokers and with more risk of fractures. In the case of AIDS, it doubles the speed at which the symptoms develop.[8]

In the age group 45 to 64, non-smokers die at the rate of 708 persons per 100,000 of the population. Smokers die at the rate of 1,329 persons per 100,000 population. Of these, heart disease accounts for 615 of the smokers' deaths but only 304 of the non-smokers' deaths. Lung cancer accounts for eighty-seven deaths for the smokers and eleven for the non-smokers. Emphysema accounts for twenty-four of the smokers' deaths and four of the non-smokers' deaths.

There are various estimates as to how much smoking shortens a life. For someone who starts smoking as a teenager, it probably shortens life by about 8 to 14 years. However, official statistics compiled in Germany indicate that the non-smoker lives 7 years longer than the average smoker of one pack a day and 14 years longer than the chain-smoker. Recent studies indicate that a 35-year-old man who smokes two packs a day reduces his life expectancy by more than 8 years.[9]

Studies on the average increase of death rates for smokers are difficult to compare because it is generally not known exactly when each smoker started to smoke, what percentage of cigarettes were high tar and nicotine or low tar and nicotine, exactly how many cigarettes were smoked, and how much side stream (passive smoke) was inhaled by the smokers and the non-smokers in the study. Hereditary weaknesses of the participants in the study are also a factor. One fact is clear, however – smoking greatly decreases the average life expectancy.

Clearly, smoking ages the smoker. It shows in the ageing of the skin and even the greying of one's hair.[10] It also increases the risk of hip fractures due to osteoporosis. The estimated cumulative risk of hip fracture in women in England was 19 per cent in smokers and 12 per cent in non-smokers to age 85; 37 per cent and 22 per cent to age 90. Among all women, one hip fracture in eight is attributable to smoking.

Limited data in men suggest a similar proportionate effect of smoking as in women.

Cigarettes kill most of their victims through heart attacks. Lung cancer claims the second greatest number and emphysema is third. It is widely believed that smoking 200,000 cigarettes (a pack a day for 25 years) is almost certain to cause one's death through lung cancer, heart attack, or by some other means. A recent New York study on women and smoking showed that for women dying of coronary heart disease (heart attacks), the average age of death for non-smokers was 67 years, for light smokers it was 55 years, and for heavy smokers, 48 years.

Since two of the major factors associated with higher death risk, nicotine and tars, can be found in differing amounts in different brands of cigarettes, smokers of low-tar, low nicotine cigarettes can reduce the expected death rate by 15 to 20 per cent of the rates of the average smoker. However, the carbon monoxide inhaled from any cigarette is approximately the same – and it is a highly damaging element to have in the blood.

Atherosclerosis (hardened arteries) in monkeys and rabbits was increased when they breathed increased carbon monoxide for 15 minutes a day for a year. Animal studies show that carbon monoxide makes the artery walls more permeable to fatty substances. This is one likely possibility to explain the high heart attack rate among smokers. Possibly more important, smoking increases the amount of cholesterol in the blood and it also reduces the amount of HDL (the good cholesterol), which thereby increases the amount of artery hardening and clogging.

Many cancers are increased by smoking. Leukaemia, a blood cancer, is increased by 30 per cent.[11]

Other cancer risks are also increased: bladder cancer (40 per cent increase), cervical cancer, oesophageal cancer (80 per cent of all cases), cancers of the stomach and colon (double the risk of non-smokers), laryngeal cancer (twenty-five times more), kidney cancers (40 per cent of all cases), mouth cancer (twenty-seven times higher) and breast cancer (75 per cent). In fact, 30 per cent of all cancers are caused by smoking.[12]

Lung cancer caused only one death in 500 in the year 1890. Today, the rate is one in fourteen. This increase is due mostly to smoking cigarettes. Since there are 50,000 times more particles in cigarette smoke than in heavy air pollution, it is easy to understand how hard it is for the lungs and the bronchial tubes to try to clean themselves of these particles.

We assume that, based on studies, cigarettes are more harmful than pipes. This was reported by the American Cancer Society. However, a recent Swedish study which dealt with 27,000 men and an equal number of women aged 18 to 69 showed that the lung cancer rates for cigarette and pipe smokers were about even – each group experienced seven times more lung cancer than non-smokers. Those who smoked both cigarettes and pipes ran 10.9 times the risk. In fact, pipe smokers who consumed as many as fifteen cigarettes a day showed twenty-nine times the risk of lung cancer. The difference may be due to the type of tobacco used and whether the pipe smokers inhaled.

Non-inhaling smokers, such as pipe and cigar smokers, tend to develop cancers of the mouth, larynx, oesophagus and on the tongue and lips. Inhalers tend to develop cancers of the lungs, the bladder and the pancreas. Lung cancer, once it has developed, is 90 per cent fatal.

The Seventh Day Adventist Church, which does not allow its members to smoke, has a very low lung cancer rate among its members, even when they live in cities where there is a great deal of air pollution. On the other hand, in Iceland, where there is very little air pollution and a high percentage of cigarette smokers, there is a high rate of lung cancer. Statistics indicate that if you stop smoking for 10 years, your chances of developing lung cancer are no greater than that of the non-smoker.

Emphysema and chronic bronchitis each year are increased by about a million new cases. Most of them are brought on by smoking. It is estimated that 99 per cent of heavy cigarette smokers (those who smoke more than one pack a day) have emphysema. In a study of 1,800 deceased people, only 10 per cent of the non-smokers had any degree of emphysema, and none had advanced emphysema.

In chronic smokers, the increased mucus in the bronchial tubes can drop into the lungs and have the same effect as water in the lungs, in effect 'drowning' the smoker because the mucus-filled alveoli (air sacs in the lungs) are not able to accept oxygen. This is caused not only by the increased mucus but also by the loss of the cilia which would have been able to eliminate some of the mucus.

Other problems caused by smoking include:

- Back pain, a common ailment among smokers and the leading cause of worker disability. The poor oxygen levels in the blood prevent the lumbar discs from being adequately oxygenated.
- Increased risk of stomach ulcers – the levels of prostaglandins, which help to protect the stomach lining, are reduced. Estimates are that there over a million more ulcers are caused by smoking.
- Increased risk of stroke (twice to six times the risk – depending on amount smoked).
- Increased diabetes risk.
- Five times more chance of developing osteoporosis in women.
- Premature ageing of the skin.
- Yellowing of teeth and fingernails.
- An increase in mouth and gum disease. Female smokers, aged 20 to 39, and male smokers, aged 30 to 59, have twice the

chance of being completely toothless from periodontal diseases than do non-smokers.
- More colds.
- More cirrhosis of the liver. The cirrhosis may be because smokers often drink more alcohol, so may be the end result of drinking and lack of food rather than smoking.
- Blindness (nicotine amblyopia) may result from the nicotine in tobacco. This is especially true for cigar and pipe smokers.

Smoking also seems to dull one's sex life, possibly because nicotine poisons the central nervous system and also interferes with the male hormone secretion. It also seems to affect male fertility. It reduces sperm production and may change the structural quality of the sperm. A recent study reported by the Soviet newspaper, *Soviet Skaya Rossiya*, reported that scientists have just completed a study showing that smoking causes chemical changes in the blood in the sex hormones. Men over 40 were most seriously affected.

GIVING UP SMOKING

Many millions of people have given up smoking. The obvious health reasons seem to be the primary motivation. However, before giving up smoking, it is a good idea to determine the type of smoker you are. Four types have been identified:

1. About 50 per cent smoke for 'positive effect'. This smoker wants a cigarette when he or she is most relaxed, such as after a meal or while drinking coffee or a liqueur. To quit, this smoker should find another pleasant habit to substitute for his or her smoking. This smoker's chances of quitting are good.
2. About 40 per cent smoke for 'negative effect'. They use smoking as a crutch – to delay doing unpleasant tasks. They smoke when ill at ease, frustrated or nervous. If they give up smoking, they will be at risk of starting again when a tense situation develops.
3. Ten per cent of smokers are 'habitual' smokers. They smoke without thinking about it, without really enjoying it. These people find it easiest to quit, as they need only be reconditioned not to smoke.
4. About 35 per cent of smokers are 'addicted'. (Some people are in more than one of the above categories.) This person feels unhappy when not able to smoke, and for them going without a cigarette can be intolerable. For this person to quit it must be done 'cold turkey'.

There are three stages in giving up smoking.

1. Contemplation

First, you must think about why you want to give up the habit. How strong is your motivation? You may have begun to think of quitting because of your increased knowledge about the many negative effects of smoking. But this may not yet have changed your attitude sufficiently. You will need a strong commitment to quitting because nicotine is an extremely addictive drug. If you do find that you have a sufficiently strong motivation, you can honestly decide to quit.

2. Quitting

There are many approaches to quitting. Some people stop by themselves, some use nicotine patches, some use educational and self-help groups. Your ability to quit will depend on how heavily you are addicted to nicotine. If you try but fail, you may be comforted to know that your chances of finally quitting increase with each attempt.

3. Maintenance

Staying nicotine-free gets easier with each passing week. During this time avoid the temptation of 'just one smoke'. It is so easy to relapse. Also, during the early stages, ask friends and family not to smoke in your presence – or leave when they light up.

If you have been a very heavy smoker and you decide to give up smoking, you may exhibit withdrawal symptoms from the depressant effects. Such effects can include: chattering teeth, uncontrollable shakes and chilling. The results of withdrawing from the stimulant effects of the release of adrenalin and norepinephrine can include depression. These usually begin within three hours and if they occur, they will be during the first day of not smoking. During this time poisons, which have been built-up by smoking, begin to affect the body. It takes between three weeks and three months for them to be totally released by the body. There will often be other discomforts such as a lack of efficiency and tenseness during the time that you are giving up smoking.

There is no magic way to give up smoking by which a person can avoid any discomfort. Here are some suggestions for methods you might use to stop the smoking habit:

- Since the major problem in giving up smoking is withdrawal from the potent chemical nicotine, it has been found that nicotine replacement methods (such as gum, lozenges and skin patches) work best. Each of these methods is about 30 per cent effective.
- Behaviour modification should help regarding the psychological reasons for smoking. You might try any or all of the following techniques:
- Do something whenever you feel the urge to smoke. You might chew gum or exercise. Try a 20-minute walk after dinner. This not only helps to keep you a little fitter, but it also occupies you at a time when you would normally be smoking.
- Don't let yourself get angry or hungry.
- Briskly rub your body with a warm washcloth to counteract the chronic vasoconstriction of the blood vessels of the skin.
- Drink at least six to eight glasses of water or juices a day. Cranberry juice is particularly good, as it facilitates the excretion of nicotine and its by-products. The high intake of fruit and fruit juices is desirable because acid urine aids in nicotine excretion. Fruit sugars also help the ex-smoker to tolerate the drop in blood sugar which occurs after nicotine withdrawal. Dried fruits can be eaten when there is a craving for a cigarette.
- Do not drink alcohol for the first 5 days of smoking abstinence because it might lessen one's determination to stop smoking. If you need to relax, try deep breathing exercises or other stress-management techniques. These may help to relieve any withdrawal anxieties.
- Coffee also increases the nicotine withdrawal symptoms, so coffee drinking should be curbed during this time.
- Hypnosis has been successfully used by some smokers. While this method has not been studied extensively, early reports indicate that it may have a success rate of between 25 and 40 per cent for the first 2-year period.

If you find you cannot stop smoking, you might consider using filters or smoking less of each cigarette, since the last part of the cigarette is the most harmful. The tobacco in the cigarette assists in filtering out some of the harmful substances, but when you smoke the last part of the cigarette you are taking in those harmful substances from the first several puffs which had been trapped on the tobacco closer to the smoker's lips.

Some people have tried to cut down their tar and nicotine intake by changing to low-tar, low nicotine cigarettes. Some use these cigarettes as they try to taper off and eventually quit the habit. Others want to continue to smoke, but at the same time lessen the negative effects on their bodies. However, if they are smoking to get the effect of the nicotine they will probably

---

Self-Test *True* or *False*

1. Nicotine is the most dangerous element in tobacco smoke. _____ _____

2. Nicotine is not much more addictive than the caffeine in coffee. _____ _____

3. The taxes on cigarettes pay all of the medical costs which smoking causes. _____ _____

4. Passive smoking inhaled by those near the smoker is less dangerous than the smoke which the smoker inhales. _____ _____

5. The illnesses caused by smokers cost the taxpayers nearly half a billion pounds per year in medical bills. _____ _____

6. The major cause of death for smokers is lung cancer. _____ _____

7. Smokeless tobacco is a safe way of using tobacco. _____ _____

8. Every year fewer people are smoking. _____ _____

9. Teenage girls take up the smoking habit more often than any other group. _____ _____

10. Stop-smoking clinics generally work. _____ _____

Answers

1. *True or false*. While nicotine is the addictive agent in tobacco smoke, the tars, carbon monoxide or any of a number of other compounds may actually be more dangerous.
2. *False*. Nicotine is highly addictive, ranking close behind crack cocaine and cocaine but more addictive than heroin.
3. *False*. Only a minor percentage of the medical costs are covered by taxes.
4. *True or false*. Since the sidestream smoke is not filtered it is more dangerous as it comes off the cigarette; however, because it is not as concentrated when it reaches the nose of the passive smoker it is less dangerous at that point.
5. *False*. Non-smokers pay over half a billion pounds a year for the illnesses of smokers.
6. *False*. Far more smokers die of tobacco-related heart disease than lung cancer.
7. *False*. A number of cancers are caused by smokeless tobacco.
8. *False*. From 1968 until the early 1990s smoking decreased. It has now levelled off.
9. *True*.
10. *False*. No technique has been developed which helps smokers to stop in a high percentage of cases. However, the more often a smoker attempts to stop the better the chances are of success. So while clinics only work for a few the first time, they work progressively more often with each new attempt by a smoker to stop.

just end up smoking more cigarettes. This is probably why the average smoker today smokes more cigarettes than did the average smoker of 1955, when high nicotine brands were popular. There is also less tobacco in cigarettes today than there was 25 years ago. The amount of tobacco required to make 1,000 cigarettes today is only 1.9lb (0.9kg) compared with the 2.7lb (1.2kg) used a quarter of a century ago. This may also have led to an increase in the number of cigarettes smoked.

Many people find that the most effective way to quit smoking is to attend a stop-smoking clinic. Most are very reasonably priced.

CHAPTER 11
Alcohol

We are all familiar with the many reasons people give for their drinking. How many of these reasons are honest and how many are rationalizations? Have we evaluated the facts before making our decision on whether or how to use alcohol? What are the advantages and what are the disadvantages of alcohol use and what are the probabilities of our abusing the drug? There are a large number of negatives, as well as a few positives, which can be said about drinking.

On the negative side, it adds useless calories, it can kill brain cells, it makes us less efficient in driving and working, and it often makes us do things we regret. On the positive side, two or three drinks a day can increase the HDL (the good cholesterol), it is a 'social lubricant' which relaxes us and can make us forget our shyness, and a good wine may complement a fine dinner.

Let's look for a moment at how alcohol can work in the body.

ABSORPTION

Absorption of alcohol occurs in the body through the tongue, stomach and small intestine. It can be slowed if the drinker has consumed a full dinner. High protein foods stay in the stomach longer and slow down the absorption of the alcohol into the bloodstream by as much as 50 per cent. Remember that all foods add calories, and each gram of

alcohol adds 7 calories. This is equivalent to 200 calories per ounce of alcohol.

The absorption of alcohol can be speeded up. Carbonation, which increases the speed with which the alcohol enters the small intestine, is a factor in increasing the speed of intoxication. Therefore, champagnes, carbonated wines or spirits mixed with soda, tonic or carbonated soft drinks speed up absorption and intoxication. Another factor which can speed alcohol absorption is the emotional set of the drinker. A person who is nervous may secrete more stomach acid, in turn increasing their ability to absorb the alcohol quickly.

Once absorbed into the blood, the liver begins to convert the alcohol into water and carbon dioxide. However, it is not done quite that simply. One of the products in the breakdown of the alcohol is acetaldehyde – which is more toxic than alcohol. This may be one of the factors in the development of the disease cirrhosis of the liver which is the bane of heavy drinkers. There is definitely a heavy toll on the liver when it is forced to oxidize great amounts of alcohol over long periods of time.

THE EFFECTS OF ALCOHOL ON THE BRAIN

The immediate effects of alcohol on the brain are substantial. While the alcohol reduces the ability of the nerves to transmit impulses, it

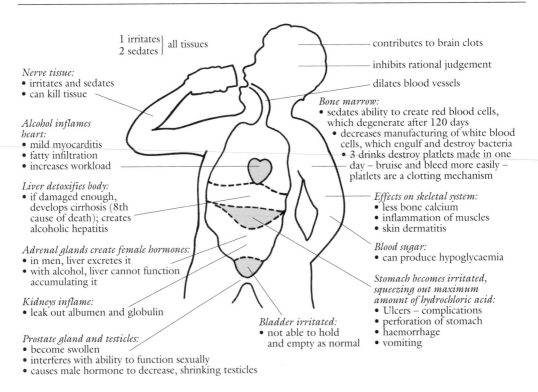

1 irritates | all tissues
2 sedates |

contributes to brain clots

inhibits rational judgement

dilates blood vessels

Nerve tissue:
• irritates and sedates
• can kill tissue

Bone marrow:
• sedates ability to create red blood cells,
  which degenerate after 120 days
• decreases manufacturing of white blood
  cells, which engulf and destroy bacteria
• 3 drinks destroy platlets made in one
  day – bruise and bleed more easily –
  platlets are a clotting mechanism

Alcohol inflames heart:
• mild myocarditis
• fatty infiltration
• increases workload

Liver detoxifies body:
• if damaged enough,
  develops cirrhosis (8th
  cause of death); creates
  alcoholic hepatitis

Effects on skeletal system:
• less bone calcium
• inflammation of muscles
• skin dermatitis

Adrenal glands create female hormones:
• in men, liver excretes it
• with alcohol, liver cannot function
  accumulating it

Blood sugar:
• can produce hypoglycaemia

Kidneys inflame:
• leak out albumen and globulin

Stomach becomes irritated,
squeezing out maximum
amount of hydrochloric acid:
• Ulcers – complications
• perforation of stomach
• haemorrhage
• vomiting

Bladder irritated:
• not able to hold
  and empty as normal

Prostate gland and testicles:
• become swollen
• interferes with ability to function sexually
• causes male hormone to decrease, shrinking testicles

Fig 7. Effects of alcohol on the human body.

also affects several neurotransmitters. Serotonin, GABA, dopamine, norepinephrine and the opioids result in the reinforcing properties of the drug.[1]

Much of the addictive effects seem to occur in the limbic system of the brain. This area includes several brain organs including the hypothalamus, the medial forebrain bundle, the front part of the cerebral cortex and other organs. In this area emotions (such as fear, rage, anxiety), memory, the stimulus for procreating and the impulse for caring of the young seem to be located.[2]

Brain cells are destroyed even in normal social drinking, whereas a heavy drinking session has been estimated to destroy as many as 10,000 brain cells. This brain cell destruction occurs for two reasons. Alcohol is a direct poison to nerve tissues. It first sedates the nerve so that it is ineffective in carrying its electrical current. In higher concentrations, it kills the nerve fibres. Since the brain has more blood flow than any other organ, alcohol is more concentrated in the brain than anywhere else.

The second reason is that alcohol has a 'blood sludging' effect on the red blood cells. They clump together and thereby slow down the blood flow. This, in turn, slows or stops the oxygen from entering the cells which need it. When this occurs in the brain, some cells die. Blood sludging can also rupture small capillaries (blood vessels) and cause small haemorrhages. (This phenomenon also occurs in about 50 different diseases, including malaria and typhoid fever.) The sludging effect of alcohol can be observed in a person's eye capillaries after having consumed just one glass of beer.

In drinking to the point of inebriation, one will incur a substantial number of small brain haemorrhages and an even larger number of plugged capillaries. Around each of these points some brain cells will die because of a lack of oxygen or because the nerve cell has been killed by the alcohol. Research on brain cells indicates that apparently our bodies cannot rebuild new brain cells in the same was as it can other types of body cells.

The average adult brain contains about seventeen billion cells, so the destruction of even a few thousand cells in a single drinking bout leaves the drinker with thinking abilities apparently intact. However, years of drinking show an accumulation of scars caused by the haemorrhages. Autopsies of heavy drinkers show that many areas of brain have shrunk where the brain cells have been destroyed.

A lesser but still important reason for the reduction of memory, including 'blackouts', is that alcohol reduces the action of the neurotransmitters and deadens the nerve fibres so that they cannot carry the impulses to the area of the brain where memory should occur. Consequently, what should be remembered, like what you did last night, cannot be remembered. The impulses which should have carried the information to the memory area of the brain have not functioned.[3] It reminds us of Ben Johnson's observation that, 'Those that talk and never think … live in the wild anarchy of drink.'

As with every upper or downer drug, there is a rebound effect as the person comes off the drug. A common example of this is when a person has been drinking, then goes to bed. Sleep generally comes rapidly but several hours later the person may wake up. The rebound has stimulated the brain and brought it into an 'upper' mode so sleep is no longer possible. Within a few more hours, after the brain has returned to normal, the person may go back to sleep. A heavy drinker will probably not recognize this factor because so much alcohol has been consumed that its effects last 8 or more hours – the time when one would normally wake up.

HANGOVERS

The 'hangover' effect, which often results from drinking, may be caused by several factors. The alcohol and other ingredients in the drinks may contribute to the unpleasant experience known as a 'hangovers'. Alcohol distends (widens) the blood vessels of the brain. Distended blood vessels are a cause of many types of headaches. Since the liver oxidizes alcohol at the rate of one-quarter to three-quarters of an ounce per hour the headache will eventually pass away as the blood vessels return to their normal sizes. The metabolism of alcohol can be speeded up somewhat by ingesting fruit sugars (fructose) which is found in honey, fresh fruits and juices. This can be done before or after imbibing.

The headache may be eased by drinking coffee. The caffeine constricts the blood vessels. One might also sit up in a dark room for a few hours. Lying down, however, would increase the flow of blood to the head. A cold compress applied to the head might also decrease blood flow.

The analgesic characteristics of aspirin may also help to relieve the headache. However, since alcohol and aspirin combined cause a chemical reaction which disintegrates the stomach lining it is not wise to take aspirin until the alcohol has left the stomach and has entered the small intestine. This might occur within 20 minutes if the stomach was empty before drinking, but might be a few hours if the stomach was full of food while the drinks were being ingested.

The dry mouth which often occurs after drinking is a result of the dehydration of the body which occurs as the alcohol is being metabolized. Drinking lots of water might combat this, but juices would be better.

The congeners (flavouring and colouring agents added to alcohol) are thought to be greatly responsible for the effects of hangover. Light coloured drinks, such as white wine, vodka and gin, are low in congeners, so should reduce the severity of a hangover. Dark liquids such as red wine, brandy, rum and whiskies are high in congeners and would, therefore, increase the effects of hangover.

ALCOHOL AND HEART DISEASE

Alcohol as a preventer of heart disease has been suggested by a number of studies recently. For example, An Australian study reports that risk is lowest among men who report one to four drinks daily on five or six days a week and among women who report one or two drinks daily on five or six days a week.[4] Red wine has been touted as being particularly beneficial. There seem to be antioxidants in the alcohol which have a positive effect on the arteries. However, while this is true it is not the whole story. The studies which prompted the findings compared Italy and France, with other European countries as well as the United States. It is true that the French and the Italians drink far more red wine than the British or the Americans and have fewer heart attacks. However, they also die from alcohol-related diseases far more than those who drink less. Cirrhosis of the liver and oesophageal cancer are three times higher among the French than the Americans. The southern Europeans also have some other dietary differences than the British and Americans. They eat much less red meat. They eat more fruits and vegetables. And they consume more fibre in their diets.

ALCOHOL AND BEHAVIOUR

The effects of alcohol on behaviour are determined, to a large degree, by what the person expects to happen or wants to happen. While alcohol depresses the ability of the brain to function normally, the behaviour which the individual exhibits may be quite varied. One person may fight, another may sleep, one may become very outgoing, another over amorous. Inhibitions are usually relaxed, which can reduce one's shyness in a social situation.

As mentioned, alcohol sedates the nerve fibres, thereby reducing the number of nerve impulses. It also works in the synapses by changing the function of several neurotransmitters. Alcohol also affects people by decreasing the amount of oxygen that the brain can utilize. A lack of oxygen in pilots has the same effect. At 9,000ft (without supplemental oxygen) one can become 'high' or drunk.

DRINKING AND DRUNKENNESS

Bertrand Russell once opined that 'Drunkenness is temporary suicide: the happiness that it brings is merely negative, a momentary cessation of unhappiness.'[5]

The amount of alcohol that a person can drink is determined, to a large degree, by their body weight. The greater the volume of blood in the person, the greater the amount of alcohol which can be dissolved in it. Also, larger people generally have larger livers with which to oxidize the alcohol. So it is the alcoholic content of the blood, not the total number of drinks, that determines one's degree of drunkenness.

If a person has been drinking for several hours, just divide the number of hours into the number of drinks plus one, to find the blood alcohol content. For example, if a 120lb (54kg) person has had eleven drinks in

Effects of Alcohol

The following chart indicates the effects of various levels of blood alcohol on behaviour. The chart is based on the blood alcohol level for a 150lb (68kg) person. A lighter person's blood alcohol level would be raised more quickly for the same amount of alcohol intake. And, conversely, a heavier person would not be affected to the same degree as the 150lb drinker.

Drink consumed	Per cent of blood alcohol	Effects
2oz 90-proof whiskey, or one bottle of beer	0.05	Dulls top layers of brain controlling moral and physical judgement. The drinker loses some inhibitions and feels less bound by minor conventions and courtesies. He feels 'on top of the world' and relaxes.
4oz 90-proof whiskey, or two bottles of beer	0.1	Further effects moral and physical control centres. Drinker becomes happier, may take some personal and physical liberties.
6oz 90-proof whiskey, or three bottles of beer	0.15	Drinker begins to stagger and sway and speech may become slurred. Reflexes are slower. He becomes careless, overconfident, acts on impulse. Depending on the individual, lax moral behaviour and/or careless driving are results of this amount of intoxication.
8oz 90-proof whiskey, or four bottles of beer	0.2	Function of lower motor and sensory areas of brain are definitely impaired. At this stage, virtually all drinkers, no matter how 'seasoned', begin to show evidence of slowed reflexes and poor judgement – both morally and physically. The drinker may begin to see double and feel sleepy.
12oz 90-proof whiskey, or six bottles of beer	0.3	There is a marked inability of gait. The drinker is obviously drunk, needs help to walk or undress, and tends to fall asleep.
14oz 90-proof whiskey, or seven bottles of beer	0.35	Affects lower, more primitive areas of the brain. Senses are dulled. Drinker falls into stupor.
14–21oz 90-proof whiskey, or eight to ten bottles of beer	0.5 to 0.6	Usually 'dead drunk'. All consciousness goes. Apart from functions of breathing and heartbeat, drinker is anaesthetized.
24–28oz 90-proof whiskey or twelve to fourteen bottles of beer	0.5 to 0.6	Puts to sleep the lowest level of brain, including centre controlling the heart and respiration. Finally the heart stops. For alcohol to cause death in this way, though, more than a quart of whiskey (or its equivalent) must be drunk in a short time.

Alcohol Impairment Chart

While the simplest guideline to remember is that for each drink consumed, wait at least 1 hour before driving – and proportionately longer for smaller people – the following chart gives more exact guidelines:

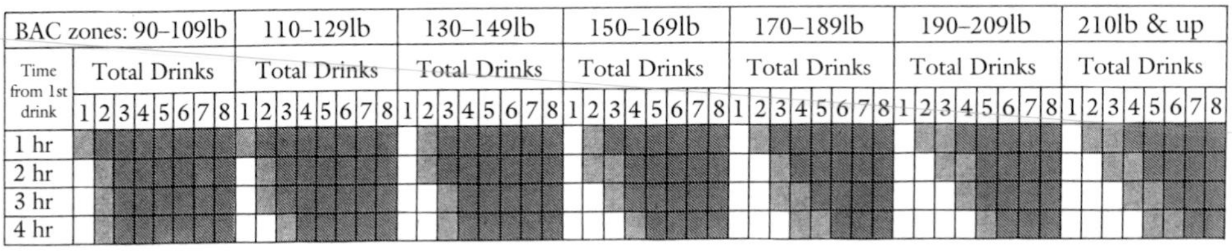

BAC zones: 90–109lb								110–129lb								130–149lb								150–169lb								170–189lb								190–209lb								210lb & up							
Time from 1st drink	Total Drinks								Total Drinks								Total Drinks								Total Drinks								Total Drinks								Total Drinks								Total Drinks							
	1	2	3	4	5	6	7	8	1	2	3	4	5	6	7	8	1	2	3	4	5	6	7	8	1	2	3	4	5	6	7	8	1	2	3	4	5	6	7	8	1	2	3	4	5	6	7	8	1	2	3	4	5	6	7	8
1 hr																																																								
2 hr																																																								
3 hr																																																								
4 hr																																																								

DUI = driving under the influence

☐ (.01%–.04%) May be DUI
▨ (.05%–.07%) Likely DUI
▓ (.08% up) Definitely DUI

Find the chart that includes your weight. Look at the total number of drinks you have had and compare that to the time shown. You can quickly tell if you are at risk of being arrested. If your BAC level is in the grey zone, your chances of having an accident are 5 times higher than if you had no drinks, and 25 times higher if your BAC falls into the black zone.

Fig 8. Blood alcohol zones.

The influence of one's blood alcohol content on one's ability to drive:

Below 0.05% – not under the influence.
0.05 to 0.10% – under the influence of alcohol, but not prima facie, evidence of being drunk.
0.10% and above is prima facie evidence of being under the influence of alcohol.

Equivalents of drinks:

12oz of beer (4% alcohol)
4oz glass of dinner wine (12% alcohol)
3oz of fortified wine (18% alcohol)
2oz of fruit brandy (25% alcohol)
1oz (shot) of distilled spirits – brandy, rum, scotch, vodka, gin, whisky (45% alcohol = 90 proof)

- A 12oz bottle of malt whisky would count as 1½ drinks (7% alcohol).

- A 3½oz strong mixed drink – martini, manhattan (30% alcohol) counts as two drinks.
- In the chart opposite, the area between the two dividing lines is the area of marginal drunkenness. The area to the right of the right line is definite drunkenness.

To determine the approximate blood alcohol of a person who has been drinking:

1. Find the person's blood alcohol level on the chart based on that person's weight and the number of drinks they have consumed.
2. Since the liver oxidizes the alcohol at the rate of about ¾ of an ounce per hour for a 150lb person (½ an ounce per hour for a 100lb person), subtract one drink per hour for people who weigh under 150lb or one-and-a-half drinks per hour for people who weigh over 150lb.
3. Count back on the chart for the approximate blood alcohol level at the present time.

Examples: A 100lb person has consumed ten drinks. If they had all been consumed in one hour, the blood alcohol level would be 0.375. But this person has been drinking steadily for 4 hours – an average of 2½ drinks per hour. Since the liver has oxidized approximately 2 ounces of alcohol (four drinks) subtract those four from the ten consumed. The person now has the equivalent of the alcohol of six drinks in his or her blood. So the blood-alcohol level would be about 0.225 – and the person would be quite drunk. But if a 200lb person had consumed six drinks over a 4-hour period (six drinks minus 4 hours times, or 1½ drinks per hour oxidized), that person would probably be legally sober.

Body weight   *Drinks*

Body weight	1	2	3	4	5	6	7	8	9	10	11	12
100lb (45kg)	.038	.075	.113	.150	.188	.225	.263	.300	.338	.375	.413	.450
120lb (54kg)	.031	.063	.094	.125	.156	.188	.219	.250	.281	.313	.344	.375
140lb (64kg)	.027	.054	.080	.107	.134	.161	.188	.241	.241	.268	.295	.321
160lb (73kg)	.023	.047	.070	.094	.117	.141	.164	.188	.211	.234	.258	.281
180lb (82kg)	.021	.042	.063	.083	.104	.125	.146	.167	.188	.208	.229	.250
200lb (91kg)	.019	.038	.056	.075	.094	.113	.131	.150	.169	.188	.206	.225
220lb (100kg)	.017	.034	.051	.068	.085	.102	.119	.136	.153	.170	.188	.205
240lb (109kg)	.016	.031	.047	.063	.078	.094	.109	.125	.141	.156	.172	.188

area of marginal
drunkeness

0.05 blood alcohol level – coordination is somewhat impaired, possibility of accident increased.
0.08 blood alcohol level is 'prima facie' evidence of being legally drunk in UK.
0.10 blood alcohol level indicates severe coordination impairment. Is evidence of being legally drunk in most countries.
0.15 blood alcohol level – legally drunk in all countries.

a 4-hour period, add one to the number of drinks (to allow for slow absorption of the first drink). We now have twelve drinks, divided by 4 hours. This is equal to three drinks per hour. The 120lb person would have a blood alcohol level of approximately 0.94 and would be very drunk.

Women are at greater risk than men from drinking for several reasons. Their bodies, on average, are smaller – so are their livers which oxidize the alcohol. They also have more fat and a lesser percentage of water than men. This allows for higher levels of blood alcohol more quickly. Women also have less of an enzyme called alcohol dehydrogenase which metabolizes some alcohol in the stomach. This factor allows more alcohol into the blood earlier.[6]

How Much is Too Much?

Various groups have set different criteria for determining what is moderate, heavy and alcoholic drinking. The Department of Health, Education and Welfare in the US has stated that a moderate drinker would drink no more than 3oz of whisky a day. This would be equivalent to three glasses of dinner wine or two pints of beer daily. On a yearly basis, it would be equivalent to 43 fifths of whisky, or 91 quarts of wine or 365 quarts of beer. (Most experts believe that two drinks per day should be the maximum amount consumed.) Your four glasses of beer a day for a year translates into 219,000 calories or 63lb (29kg) of body fat, and your half bottle of wine (three glasses) contains 99,635 calories which becomes 28lb (13kg) of fat on your hips. Beer gets about 65 per cent of its calories from the alcohol and wine gets about 85 per cent of its calories from the alcohol.

Reducing the Amount of Alcohol Consumed

This can be done in a number of ways. You can switch to other beverages. Fruit juices may be a possibility, although they also contain a number of calories. If you really like the taste of beer, there are some alcohol-free beers which taste just as good as beer. (There are also some that don't taste at all like beer.) Sparkling cider can replace wine or champagne. Mixed drinks of fruit punch are quite tasty. You might even add a spirit-flavoured substance, such as a rum flavoured cake additive, to make the drink taste more alcoholic. Alcohol has no taste. A drink has only the residual taste of whatever it was fermented or distilled from; your imagination can go a long way in making drinks with the 'romance' of alcohol but not its negative effects.

Wine has not yet been successfully dealcoholized. When the alcohol is removed from wine, the esters, which give it its fragrance, are also removed. Most dealcoholized wines are a combination of the wine, grape juice made from the same grape, and additional water. They taste much sweeter than the original wine and do not have the same fragrance. Experiments are now being conducted which, if successful, will remove the alcohol without removing the flavours.

ADDICTION TO ALCOHOL – ALCOHOLISM

Obviously you cannot be fit if you are an alcoholic. You can exercise and perhaps have your body in pretty good shape, but your total mind-body fitness cannot be complete.

There is a problem in defining alcoholism. Dr E.M. Jellinek, one of the pioneers in the study of alcoholism, defined it as 'a progressive disease characterized by uncontrollable drinking'. He suggested that there may be five types of alcoholics:

1. The person who is psychologically dependent on the drug and drinks to relieve psychic pain, such as: self-consciousness, fear or boredom – or to overcome an inhibition.
2. The person who drinks to relieve physical pain.
3. The person who is physically, but not psychologically, dependent. This type is common in France.
4. The person who is both psychologically and physically dependent. This type is quite common in the United States.
5. The binge drinker who drinks large amounts at one time but does not usually drink between binges. This is more common in the Scandinavian countries and Russia.

Alcoholics Anonymous defines alcoholism as 'an allergy of the body with an obsession of the mind'. The World Health Organization defines it as 'any form of drinking which in its extent goes beyond the traditional and customary dietary use of alcohol'. Other definitions of alcoholism are when the drug interferes with work, important life tasks or personal relationships. The simplest, and perhaps the most accurate definition comes from a Catholic priest, Father Joseph Martin, a recovering alcoholic, and one of the world's

---

Signs of Alcoholism

1. Drinking in secret, to keep others from knowing how much is being drunk.
2. Overriding concern with drinking. Drinking becomes more important than people.
3. Drinking the first few drinks fast to 'get high' quickly.
4. Development of guilt feelings because of the drinking:

   a. Avoiding talking about alcohol, usually for fear that the excess drinking will be criticized.
   b. Rationalizing drinking behaviour; one can always give a reason for drinking (to celebrate, to drown one's sorrows, because it is Friday).
   c. Protecting one's ego by being important, leaving large tips, buying drinks for strangers and so on.
   d. Often feeling remorse from the guilt about drinking.

5. May observe periods of total abstinence to prove that one really doesn't need alcohol. The alcoholic wants to leave the impression that it is possible to 'take it or leave it.'
6. May change drinking patterns, changing the types of drinks or the times or places which had been usual occasions for drinking.

7. In extreme cases the alcoholic may neglect everything except drinking and may become very introverted.
8. Financial problems or shame may affect the family of the alcoholic making them withdraw from normal social situations.
9. Hiding bottles of alcohol so that the supply will not run out.
10. Alcoholics may feel a great deal of self pity or resentment because of imaginary injustices they have suffered.
11. Neglecting nutrition in favour of drinking.
12. Sex drive decreases. This sometimes makes alcoholics accuse their spouse of infidelity.
13. Morning drinking.
14. Drinking to avoid the withdrawal symptoms. Since alcohol can be an addictive 'downer', the absence of alcohol can develop such symptoms as shaking and hallucinations in the alcoholic.
15. Drinking during working hours and missing work because of alcohol.
16. Lessening of tolerance for alcohol. Since the liver loses its ability to oxidize alcohol as liver tissue is destroyed by the alcohol, the alcohol stays in the body longer. It therefore takes less alcohol to get drunk and the effects of the alcohol are increased and prolonged.
17. Brain damage, loss of memory and personality changes.

---

great teachers about the disease: 'if alcohol causes problems, it is one'.

ALCOHOL AND PHYSICAL FITNESS

Alcohol affects nearly every body organ. Everyone knows that it affects the brain. But it also affects the heart, pancreas, mouth and oesophagus, and nearly every other organ. It is most likely to cause problems where you have a hereditary weakness. So if your heart is susceptible you might develop severe problems, perhaps even fatal ones, if you drink after exercising.

Some marathon runners drink beer during the race. This is counter-productive. As good as that bitter bubbly drink tastes, it is not giving your tissues the water they need. All alcohol

Self-Test

Questions About Your Drinking	*Yes*	*No*

1. Do you occasionally drink heavily after a disappointment, a quarrel or when the boss gives you a hard time?   _____ _____
2. When you have trouble or feel under pressure, do you always drink more heavily than usual?   _____ _____
3. Have you noticed that you are able to handle more alcohol than when you first started drinking?   _____ _____
4. Have you ever woken up on the 'morning after' and discover that you could not remember part of the evening before, even though your friends tell you that you did not 'pass out'?   _____ _____
5. When drinking with other people, do you try to have a few extra drinks when others will not notice it?   _____ _____
6. Are there certain occasions when you feel uncomfortable if alcohol is not around?   _____ _____
7. Have you recently noticed that when you begin drinking you are in more of a hurry to get to the first drink than you used to be?   _____ _____
8. Do you sometimes feel a little guilty about your drinking?   _____ _____
9. Are you secretly irritated when your family or friends discuss your drinking?   _____ _____
10. Have you recently noticed an increase in the frequency of your memory blackouts?   _____ _____
11. Do you often find that you wish to continue drinking after your friends say they have had enough?   _____ _____
12. Do you usually have a reason for the occasions when you drink heavily?   _____ _____
13. When you are sober, do you often regret things you have done or said while drinking?   _____ _____
14. Have you tried to switch brands or follow different plans in order to control your drinking?   _____ _____
15. Have you often failed to keep the promises you have made to yourself about controlling or cutting down on your drinking?   _____ _____
16. Have you ever tried to control your drinking by switching jobs or moving to a new location?   _____ _____
17. Do you try to avoid family or close friends while you are drinking?   _____ _____
18. Are you having an increasing number of financial or work problems?   _____ _____
19. Do more people seem to be treating you unfairly without good reason?   _____ _____
20. Do you eat very little or irregularly when you are drinking?   _____ _____
21. Do you sometimes have the 'shakes' in the morning and find out that it helps to have a little drink?   _____ _____
22. Have you recently noticed that you cannot drink as much as you once did?   _____ _____
23. Do you sometimes stay drunk for several days at a time?   _____ _____
24. Do you sometimes feel very depressed and wonder if life is worth living?   _____ _____
25. Sometimes after periods of drinking, do you see or hear things that are not there?   _____ _____
26. Do you feel terribly frightened after you have been drinking heavily?   _____ _____

If you answered 'yes' to any of the questions, you have some of the symptoms that may indicate alcoholism. 'Yes' answers to several of the questions indicate the following stages of alcoholism:

Questions 1–8 Early stage; 9–21 Middle stage; 22–26 Beginning of the final stage.

(From the US National Council on Alcoholism)

uses the body's water to help to break it down so the beer is taking, rather than giving, water. Save the beer until well after the race. In a study done at the University Medical School, Forresterhill, Aberdeen,[7] it was found that the more alcohol that was consumed, the greater the amount of urine produced and the less fluid was found in the blood.

Since alcohol depresses the central nervous system, it impairs mental and physical skills and decreases athletic performance. Even social use of alcohol the day before an event may affect performance. Skills that are especially affected by alcohol are accuracy, balance, steadiness, reaction time, complex and fine motor coordination, visual tracking and information processing. Strength and power, muscle endurance and aerobic endurance are also diminished with alcohol use.[8] Another study[9] found that runners who drank alcohol before a treadmill run had higher heart rates, lower blood sugar levels, and more trouble finishing their runs compared with runners who had drunk non-alcoholic drinks.

It has been thought that in low doses, alcohol can help to reduce anxiety and tremors, which is why some athletes competing in such sports as archery and shooting, where a steady hand is helpful, have used alcohol as a performance aid. However, they are actually hurting their performance because alcohol decreases hand–eye coordination, judgment and tracking. The International Olympic Committee has banned alcohol use in these events. So alcohol does not seem to have a place in any performance activities in which physical fitness or coordination is a factor.

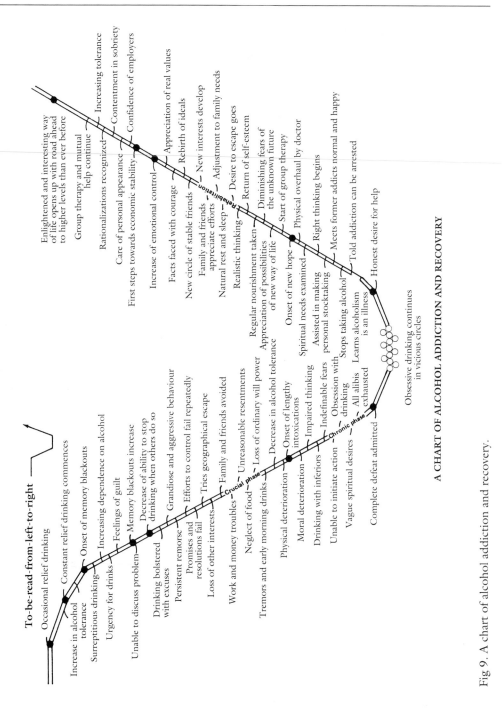

A CHART OF ALCOHOL ADDICTION AND RECOVERY

Fig 9. A chart of alcohol addiction and recovery.

CHAPTER 12
Physical Fitness for Endurance

Fitness means that the individual is able to perform the normal daily activities with adequate energy and still have the vigour to perform additional activities. If a person can finish daily chores such as school work, housekeeping or gardening, and return home with the energy necessary to play tennis, jog, or work on a hobby, a minimal level of fitness has been achieved. The higher one's level of fitness, the greater will be the reserve of energy throughout the day.

The physical effects of exercising for endurance (aerobic fitness) are many. It benefits every body organ. The major emphases of exercise have correctly been focused on the benefits to the heart and circulatory system, but it should also be noted that the bones and ligaments, digestive and excretory systems, the lymphatic and respiratory systems all benefit.

The well-conditioned person is not only able to ward off infectious diseases and cancers better than the poorly conditioned person, but the chances of developing heart disease, strokes, diabetes and other types of degenerative and chronic diseases are also lessened.

The mental effects of exercise have long been observed by athletes and physiologists of exercise. People exercising regularly generally have shown higher than average levels of social maturity, self-confidence and intellectual efficiency. The question is – did the athletic activity actually develop these qualities or were they already present in the person and perhaps were instrumental in the decision to become an athlete?

A study at Purdue University showed that untrained middle-aged university employees significantly improved their mental outlooks during the duration of a specially designed fitness programme of callisthenics and jogging. Results of the study showed that statistically significant positive changes had occurred. The areas of self-assurance, stability and imagination were all greatly improved in the test subjects.

The circulation of blood to the brain during exercise aids in making one more alert. The physical activity during exercise can also allow one to take out aggressions on inanimate objects, becoming more relaxed in the process. When people hit a tennis ball or pound the pavement while jogging, they may be unconsciously taking out frustrations which might otherwise be directed at a boss, a spouse or a neighbour.

There is a substance called catecholamine which is essential in several brain chemicals which help to transmit messages in the brain. One of the essential precursors for this brain chemical is called tyrosine hydroxylase (TH). TH decreases with age and may be a factor in mental changes and problems which can occur with age. The Geriatric Research, Education and Clinical Center of the Department of Veterans Affairs Medical Center in Gainesville, Fl, has done a study with rats which showed that exercise reduced the loss of TH. If this proves to be the same for humans we may have yet another reason for the benefits of exercise.[1]

Benefits of Aerobic Exercise

- An increase in the number of blood vessels. When this occurs in the heart, it increases one's chances of avoiding or surviving a heart attack.
- Control of body fat. One-half hour of proper exercise daily will keep off (or take off) 26lb (12kg) per year.
- An increase in the basal metabolism for several hours after exercising, which may take off additional pounds.
- An increase in HDLs (the good blood cholesterols).
- A strengthening of the diaphragm, the major muscle used in breathing.
- An improved immunity system to fight off degenerative and infectious diseases.
- Stronger bones and connective tissue.
- A reduction in minor aches, pains, stiffness and soreness.
- Increased productivity.
- A reduction in chronic fatigue.
- An increased ability to relax and to sleep well.
- An increase in endorphins in the brain (if the exercise is sufficiently long), making one feel exhilarated.
- Improved digestion and bowel function.
- Increased mental capabilities (such as increased alertness) due to an increase in oxygen to the brain.
- Increased muscle tone.
- Increased self-esteem.
- Increased creativity and imagination.
- Decreased muscle tension and stress.
- Decreased menstrual symptoms and menstrual cramps.
- Decreased labour pain and faster recovery time from giving birth.
- Lower resting heart rate from a larger stroke volume.
- Lower resting blood pressure.
- Increased life expectancy and better quality of life.

Another reason for exercising aerobically is that we look better when we exercise effectively. And when we look good, we feel good. This aesthetic value of exercise, usually combined with some diet changes, is a reason that we see so many people of all ages exercising before the summer beach season.

The benefits of exercise to a society and its economy have been recognized by the governments of China, Japan and Russia. In those countries 'exercise breaks' often take the place of coffee or tea breaks. Many US companies are developing exercise programmes to increase the physical and mental health of their employees and to increase their longevity. Such programmes have been shown to increase job performance by making the people less prone to make errors, more able to produce and less likely to miss work.

A number of people participate in Master's competition. This competition usually begins in the 30 to 40 year age range and can go up to 100! There are competitions in running, swimming, orienteering, rowing, cycling, volleyball and nearly every other sport one can imagine. In a Canadian study on Masters' participants during the 7-year follow up of the 750 respondents (aged 40 to 81 with an average of 58), far fewer than expected had developed a serious illness. Most had given up smoking before or during their training period. Only 2.9% still smoked, while 32.8% were former smokers. The participants were shown to have become more interested in their health than the general population, as witnessed by their increased use of seat belts when driving and a greater propensity to see a doctor if something seemed wrong. And, more important, their outlooks were happier and their lives seem more fulfiling.

The advantages of exercise apply equally to women and men. The old notions that exercise is unfeminine have been dispelled. The fascinatingly feminine Olga Korbut of the Russian gymnastic team captured the hearts of the world in the 1972 Olympics. Then Nadia Comaneci of Romania did it again in 1976. Then Greta Weitz, multiple marathon winner from Norway, did it. In fact, women champions in every field have shown the advantages of physical fitness. It has finally been recognized by the medical profession and the Olympic Committee that women can do anything that men can do. This idea has filtered to the general population where we now see women running, lifting weights, playing football, and water polo in addition to the sports they have traditionally participated in – swimming, tennis, gymnastics and riding.

The fears of some, that women who exercise would become too muscular, have been proved to be unfounded. The fact is that exercise aids in slimming the figure to conform to the bone structure of the natural female anatomy. Exercise can flatten the abdomen, remove excess fat, firm the muscles and assist in the development of a more attractive posture. Proper exercise can also aid in shaping the body to more desirable dimensions.

It is now recognized that women, because of their larger fat stores, can have greater endurance than can men. The marathon is a 26-mile, 385yd (42.2km) race. Women continue to reduce the margin between themselves and the faster men. However, in the supermarathon events women's times generally equal men's times at the point of 35 to 43 miles (56 to 70km). They then become faster than the men. According to studies at the University of Cape Town, this is probably due to lighter body weight, more fat stores and a better ability to convert fat into sugars for energy.[2]

A study in Minnesota of 40,000 women aged 55 to 69 showed that as little as one day a week of exercise significantly reduced their death rates. But the more physical activity they undertook, and the more vigorous it was, the lower their death rates.[3] Good physical condition can aid women in reducing most of the diseases of ageing.

Exercise also helps to relieve the menstrual discomforts which women often experienced. The high body heat and increased circulation which occur during exercise aid in relieving the congestion of blood in the uterus, a major cause of discomfort.

A Harvard University study found that female runners produced a less potent form of oestrogen than their non-exercising counterparts. This was held to be a factor in the 50 per cent reduction of expected cases of breast and cervical cancers and a 65 per cent reduction in a type of diabetes which is more common among women than men.

AGE AND EXERCISE

Age is a factor when it comes to choosing the type and amount of exercise that one should do. A person who has been exercising regularly will be 'younger' than a person who has not been exercising. That is, the condition of the person's body, its biological age, will be less than that expected for that person's chronological age. So while for the average person their conditioning level (scientifically called the VO_2 max) reduces by about 1 per cent per year after the age of 25, a well-conditioned person can slow or even reverse that normal condition of ageing. Staying fit can cut that figure in half or even reverse it.[4]

If someone has not done much exercise, the body may appear older than it really is. The bones may be softer, the blood pressure higher, the amount of artery hardening greater, the blood supply less, the digestive processes slower, the muscle cells reduced through degeneration, and many other such factors which we associate with age may be present. But if that same person were to begin an effective exercise programme, those results of ageing can be slowed, stopped, or even reversed.

Osteoporosis (porous bones), which afflicts many older women and some thin men, can be prevented or reversed by weight-bearing exercise. Walking or running, weightlifting or callisthenics can all prevent its development. Swimming, while an effective endurance exercise, does not prevent the disease because the water, not the person's body, supports the weight.

People can continue to exercise throughout their lives. Evidence indicates that such exercise should help to prolong life because it keeps the body younger. A few years ago, a San Francisco man made headlines. He was over 100 years old but he ran 7 miles each day – on his way to work as a waiter. When he finally retired from that job, at 103, he took a job working in a gym.

You may have heard of the Abkasian peasants in Asia who live to be very old. Their longevity is attributed to exercise. Not long ago, one of the boys from this area was accepted into medical school. After his graduation, he took his mother to live with him in the city, thinking that she deserved a rest in her old age. Although she had been healthy when she arrived, her health failed rapidly in the city. When she returned to the farm and working in the fields, her health returned to normal.

Exercise can make you feel better and live longer, no matter when you begin your programme. If you begin when you are young and continue the programme, you may add years to your life – and life to your years. But you are never too old to begin. After all, exercise may be the next best thing to the fountain of youth.

PHYSICAL FITNESS

The elements of physical fitness should be understood by anyone considering pursuing an effective path towards fitness. These elements are:

- Flexibility – the ability to move the joints of the body through a wide range of motion.
- Strength – the ability to lift a weight one time.
- Endurance or stamina – the ability to perform a certain task for a long period of time.
- Agility – the ability of the body to exhibit coordinated muscular movements.

Everyone should possess a minimum acceptable level of endurance, adequate strength to live their chosen lifestyle and sufficient flexibility to be able to move freely and to have an acceptably good posture.

CARDIO-VASCULAR ENDURANCE

Endurance (stamina) is the ability of the body to continue work or exercise over a long period of time. Stamina is developed by exercises which make the heart beat fast – particularly for at least 30 minutes. This is the most important aspect of physical fitness.

Most of us have the minimum level of flexibility and strength to live our lives effectively. We generally have enough sugar in our blood or fat on our bodies to give us fuel for energy. However, we often lack the ability to exercise at a level beyond that which is our norm.

Those who have developed cardiovascular (heart-blood) or cardiopulmonary (heart-lung) endurance have trained their bodies to use oxygen efficiently. Since oxygen is just as important in developing energy as is blood sugar, but it cannot be stored like sugar, the ability to use oxygen effectively must be developed.

Very few people function at even the most minimal fitness levels. Yet proper exercise, for as

---

Self-Test

Answer YES or NO to each question.

1. I climb stairs rather than take the lift whenever possible. _____
2. I know my resting pulse rate. _____
3. I know my blood pressure. _____
4. I know that aerobic exercise at least three times a week will reduce my
    heart attack risk. _____
5. I do aerobic exercise (swimming, running, aerobics, and so on.) at least three
    times per week. _____
6. I know my target heart rate for aerobic exercise. _____
7. I do abdominal curl-ups at least 3 days a week. _____
8. I do exercises for my lower back at least three times per week. _____
9. I believe that exercise will improve my mental health. _____
10. I know that aerobic exercise is one of the best things I can do to maintain my
    desired weight. _____

Nine to ten 'Yes' answers indicate that you are quite aware of your physical fitness and its importance.
Seven to eight 'Yes' answers indicate a fair understanding of the principles of physical fitness.
Five to six 'Yes' answers indicate that you need to improve your knowledge and behaviour in the physical fitness area.

---

little as 30 minutes each day, can make one's body function better, control obesity, reduce mental tensions and reduce one's chances of heart and blood circulation problems. For one's physical and mental health, for a better chance of a longer and happier life, there is probably no better investment of one's time than in a daily dose of proper endurance exercise.

Most national medical associations have now taken the position that, 'Exercise is the most significant factor contributing to the health of the individual.' Study after study indicates that proper endurance exercise is a major factor in increasing one's chances of living a longer life. A study of over 17,000 British executives showed that those who exercised vigorously had only one-third the risk of developing a fatal disease during middle age compared to light exercisers or non-exercisers.

The effects of endurance exercise on the circulatory system are:

• The heart enlarges, enabling it to pump more blood in less time to the muscles and tissues that need it. The enlarged heart beats slower than a normal heart when resting; it has a longer rest period between each beat.
• The red blood cells become more numerous. These are the cells which carry oxygen from the lungs to the muscles and other tissues of the body. The increase in these blood cells enables each beat of the heart to carry more oxygen to the tissues.
• The number of blood vessels being used in the muscles is increased. This gives the muscles more capacity for using the oxygen which is brought to them in the blood.

The heart is really a double pump. One pump (the right heart) receives 'used' blood which has just come from the body after delivering nutrients and oxygen to the body tissues. The blood is received into the right atrium (Latin

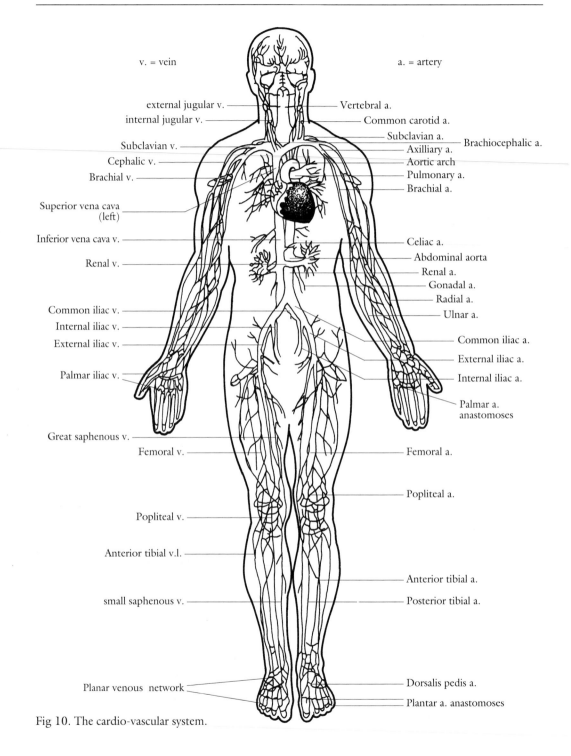

v. = vein   a. = artery

external jugular v.
internal jugular v.
Vertebral a.
Common carotid a.
Subclavian a.
Brachiocephalic a.
Axilliary a.
Aortic arch
Pulmonary a.
Brachial a.

Subclavian v.
Cephalic v.
Brachial v.

Superior vena cava (left)

Inferior vena cava v.
Renal v.

Celiac a.
Abdominal aorta
Renal a.
Gonadal a.
Radial a.
Ulnar a.

Common iliac v.
Internal iliac v.
External iliac v.

Common iliac a.
External iliac a.
Internal iliac a.

Palmar iliac v.

Palmar a. anastomoses

Great saphenous v.
Femoral v.
Femoral a.

Popliteal a.

Popliteal v.

Anterior tibial v.l.

Anterior tibial a.

small saphenous v.
Posterior tibial a.

Planar venous network

Dorsalis pedis a.
Plantar a. anastomoses

Fig 10. The cardio-vascular system.

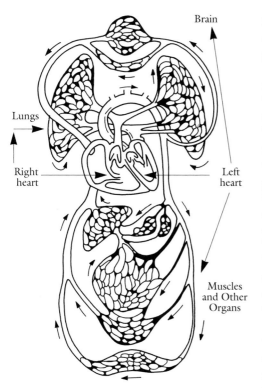

Fig 11. Representation of the cardio-vascular system.

for room). It is then pumped into the right ventricle where the next heartbeat pumps this dark, bluish red blood to the lungs, where the blood gets rid of a waste gas (carbon dioxide) and picks up a fresh supply of oxygen which turns it a bright red again. The second pump (the left heart) receives this 'reconditioned' blood from the lungs in the left atrium. The next beat pushes the newly oxygenated blood into the heavily muscled left ventricle. The next beat pumps the blood out through the great trunk-artery (aorta) to be distributed by smaller arteries to all parts of the body.

The heart can enlarge normally, because it has been forced to work hard to pump the blood of a person who exercises for long periods of time. Swimmers, basketball players and long distance runners usually have such enlarged hearts. This 'normal' enlargement is generally considered to be good.

However, abnormal heart enlargement is found in many people for various reasons. The hearts of these people have been forced to beat rapidly for reasons other than exercise. The heart of an obese person will have to beat many more times each day just to pump blood through the excess fat of that person. Some people have abnormally enlarged hearts because their heart valves do not function efficiently, or because their arteries are clogged and narrowed so that the heart must push the blood at a much higher pressure to get the blood to the organs and muscles. The previously mentioned heart valve damage can also cause the heart to enlarge due to the extra work that it is forced to do.

A normally enlarged heart will beat slower than normal as it enlarges. An abnormally enlarged heart will generally continue to beat relatively fast since it has enlarged because of extreme stresses. Its enlargement would allow more blood to be pumped with each beat, but because of the great demands of the body (such as in obesity) or in the heart's inefficiency (such as in damaged valves), enlargement is not enough. The heart must therefore continue to beat at a relatively fast rate.

The Pulse Rate

The pulse rate is the number of heart beats per minute. The average heartbeats seventy to eighty times per minute while a person is at rest. But the lower the pulse rate, the better conditioned the person is. Some athletes have pulse rates in the thirties. A pulse rate of fifty would be very good for the average person. A former Swedish tennis great had a pulse rate of twenty-eight. This was achieved because of the way he practised, continually running while hitting for several hours every day.

111

There are several methods of finding your pulse rate. First, you must find an artery which is near to the skin. The most common places are: just inside the muscle on the left side of the neck; at the base of the neck just inside the collar bone, on the inside of the wrist about 2in (5cm) below the base of the thumb, or directly over the heart. Place the fingers, not the thumb, of one hand on one of these spots. If your fingers are at the correct place, you will feel a throbbing. Each throb is a pulsation of blood from the heart. Count the number of beats for one minute. Or count the number of beats for 15 seconds and multiply by four. This will give you your resting pulse rate in beats per minute. If you are exercising you might count for 6 seconds then multiply by ten to get your pulse rate.

A heart which beats at seventy beats per minute has half a second to fill with blood. This resting phase is called the diastolic period. If the pulse rate is increased to 120 beats per minute the resting phase is reduced to a quarter of a second. In spite of the shorter resting phase, the heart still remains functional to about 160 beats per minute. At that point, the resting phase may be so short that the right atrium of the heart cannot fill completely with blood, and each beat may pump less blood.

Even though the resting phase of the heart is diminished, there are other things which happen to keep the heart efficient. The blood pressure increases, which pushes more blood into the heart. The veins may be being massaged by the muscles as the muscles contract, which aids in the more rapid return of blood to the heart. The blood becomes more acidic due to the lactic acid formed in the muscles as a result of the use of sugars for energy. This acidic quality makes the haemoglobin in the red blood cells more able to pick up the oxygen in the lungs. These factors enable the heart to pump four to ten times as much blood during heavy exercise as during rest.

The well-conditioned person's heart gets more resting periods than does the heart of the person in average condition. If a person's heart were to beat twenty times less per minute (for example, sixty rather than eighty beats per minute), it would save nearly 10,000 beats during a night's sleep and nearly 30,000 beats in a 24-hour day. It would get 18 days per year more rest than the heart with the higher pulse rate.

The heart is a very strong pump. Each day it pumps about 13 tons of blood. Each minute it pumps the total volume of the body's blood through the circulatory system. During heavy exercise, it may pump the entire volume of the blood of the body nine times each minute. That's a lot of work for a 12oz organ.

Red Blood Cells

Red blood cells carry the oxygen from the lungs to the body tissues, by means of an iron compound called haemoglobin. These red blood cells are 1/3,500 of an inch in diameter. They are formed in the bone marrow and live about 3 months. When red cells are destroyed, the body reclaims most of the iron and uses it to form new red cells. If one's diet is deficient in iron, it will probably result in anaemia (a lack of red cells).

The more blood and red cells present in each unit of blood, the greater the oxygen-carrying capacity of the blood. If a person lives high above sea level, the body's need for oxygen increases. This is because the air at high altitudes is less dense, so there is less oxygen per cubic foot of air. The body then manufactures more red blood cells so that a greater proportion of the oxygen in the air is absorbed. The Aymara Indians of the Andes Mountains have an average red cell blood count of eight million per cubic centimetre of blood. The average person at sea level has a red cell count of about 4.5 million. Strenuous exercise and high altitude living both have the same effect on the red cell count. As the body's need for oxygen increases, the red blood cells increase to accommodate that need – if the diet contains sufficient iron.

Exercise also increases the total amount of blood in the body. The average person can increase the total amount of blood by 10 to 20 per cent during 10 weeks of effective endurance training. This can increase the blood volume by up to 2 quarts. Well-trained athletes may have over 40 per cent more blood circulating in their bodies compared to average people. This means that the heart does not have to pump as often to get the necessary oxygen to the muscles and other tissues because each spoonful of blood carries more red cells and consequently more oxygen.

The condition of the muscles is another factor in one's endurance. Only the muscles which are specifically involved in the activity gain endurance. The legs of a long-distance runner or cyclist and the chest and upper back muscles of a swimmer will have developed changes when they become well conditioned. The number of small blood vessels (capillaries) being used by the muscle will increase so that more blood will be able to circulate through the muscle. This allows more oxygen and blood sugars to be available for energy.

HOW MUCH EXERCISE DO I NEED?

The original work of Dr Ken Cooper in his book *Aerobics* required several exercise sessions each week at a fairly high level of intensity. Later, the American College of Sports Medicine adopted and refined a more stringent programme. (This will be discussed in the next section.) However, the work of Dr Steven Blair, of Dr Cooper's Institute for Aerobic Research in Texas, indicates that if your objective for exercising is merely living longer, you can exercise at a lower level of intensity. Dr Blair has used research based on 25,000 people followed for many years to develop his theory.

The 'minimal exercise requirement' allows a person to build up his or her exercise during a day. The 'maximum fitness exercise programme' requires a person to do 20 to 30 minutes work at one session to achieve maximum results. Dr Blair's minimum requirement would allow a person to add the exercise done in a day to achieve the minimum 30 minutes. So, if you walk 10 minutes in the morning, climb stairs for a total of 1 minute during the day, garden for 20 minutes, then ride a bicycle for 10 minutes in the evening you would have totalled at least 41 minutes of exercise during the day. Just 30 minutes is enough to increase your chances of living longer.[5]

Dr Blair's analyses of his 25,000 subjects over the years has led to a large number of scientific articles and has changed our thinking relative to what is a minimal work out for extending our life spans.

On the other side of the exercise spectrum, work at Dr. Cooper's Center indicates that if you exercise with some intensity, which is the message of this book, you need not exercise more than a half hour in order to get many of the benefits necessary for maximum heart disease protection. Exercising up to 60 minutes per day gives additional benefits. More than 60 minutes a day at a high pulse rate does not seem to reduce the risk of heart disease. More than 60 minutes would burn more calories and contribute to weight loss. It would also reduce the risk of some types of diabetes. However the wear and tear on the joints from running might be a negative risk factor for too much jogging. So more than an hour a day of exercise should only be done if it is enjoyable and does not cause any physical pain.[6]

A British study indicates that you need to burn 7.5 calories per pound per hour in order to gain improved health.[7] An American study[8]

Metabolic Rates

Often today in scientific research the term MET (metabolic rate at rest) is used. Researchers use multiples of that resting rate to show how much more energy is being expended during the exercise. It is equal to about 80 per cent of the number of calories (kilocalories).

For the average man 143lb (65kg):

Exercise level	Number of kilocalories per minute	METS
Resting/sleeping	1.25	1
Light	2.0–4.9	1.6–3.9
Moderate	5.0–7.4	4.0–5.9
Heavy	7.5–9.9	6.0–7.9
Very heavy	10.0–12.4	8.0–9.9
Extremely heavy	12.5+	10.0+

For the average woman 121lb (55kg):

Exercise level	Number of kilocalories per minute	METS
Resting/sleeping	1.25	1
Light	1.5–3.4	1.2–2.7
Moderate	3.5–5.4	2.8–4.3
Heavy	5.5–7.4	4.4–5.9
Very heavy	7.5–9.4	6.0–7.5
Extremely heavy	9.5+	7.6+

To determine your own number of kilocalories per minute:

Men 143 (for the average man) divided by 65 × your weight.

Women 121 (for the average woman) divided by 55 × your weight.

suggests a weekly output of 2,000 calories in exercise in order to achieve a minimal level of fitness. This would require 5 hours of exercise per week with an expenditure of 8 calories per minute.

So to determine how much you should exercise depends on what you want:

- If you want to extend your life some and feel better, do 30 minutes of increased exercise each day – not necessarily continuously;
- If you want a higher level of fitness with a greatly lessened heart attack risk, do 30 minutes of continuous exercise at 65 to 90 per cent of your maximal heart rate (220 minus your age).
- If you want still more benefits, exercise up to an hour at the higher heart rate.
- If you want to lose fat, exercise longer but at a much lower pulse rate.

EXERCISING FOR BETTER AEROBIC FITNESS

Effective aerobic exercise, according to the American College of Sports Medicine (ACSM) report of 1990, requires that aerobic exercise be done three to five times per week for 20 to 60 minutes each session at an intensity of 60–90 per cent of maximum heart rate or 50 to 85 per cent of maximum oxygen consumption. (In addition, ACSM recommends the inclusion of a strength training programme for overall health benefits.)

To determine your target heart rate zone (where your heart rate should be while exercising to increase cardiorespiratory fitness), you must first determine your maximal heart rate. This is done by subtracting your age from 220. Then, you can determine the limits of your intensity by multiplying your

Evaluation of Daily Calorific Requirements

Evaluate your daily caloric expenditure over several days to get an idea of your activity level. The values below are in calories per pound per hour. Record your activity level below:

Calories per hour × Weight in lbs × Number of hours = Total calories used

	Calories per hour	× Weight in lbs	× Number of hours	= Total calories used
Sleeping or lying in bed	0.12	× _____	× _____	= _____
Sitting (reading, on computer, bathing, eating, etc)	0.17	× _____	× _____	= _____
Standing (washing, shaving, cooking, etc	0.26	× _____	× _____	= _____
Light work (housework, driving, mechanics, slow walking)	0.38	× _____	× _____	= _____
Faster work (table tennis, volleyball, sailing or canoeing, golf)	0.55	× _____	× _____	= _____
Heavier manual labour (carpentry, machine operation, plumbing, shovelling snow)	0.64	× _____	× _____	= _____
Active sports (downhill skiing, tennis, badminton, dancing, fast walking, slow jogging)	0.77	× _____	× _____	= _____
Very heavy exercise (cross-country skiing, running fast, basketball, football, digging, sawing with hand saw)	0.90	× _____	× _____	= _____
			_____	_____
			Total 24 hours	*Calories used in a day*

maximal heart rate by between .6 and .9. (The higher number is for better conditioned people.) For instance, if you are 50 years old, then your maximal heart rate is 220–50 = 170. To determine your minimal target heart rate, multiply $170 \times .6 = 102$ beats per minute. For the top of your target heart rate zone, multiply $170 \times .9 = 153$ beats per minute. Beginners should start at the low end of the target heart rate range, and slowly increase their

exercising heart rate as their body adapts to the increased physical demands of exercise.

Exercise physiologists use another measure to determine cardiorespiratory fitness – the VO_2 max. It determines the amount of oxygen which a body can use to develop energy while exercising. (The maximum amount of oxygen used (VO_2 max) is the number of millilitres (ml) of oxygen (O_2) per kilogram of body weight per minute.) Males generally have about a 20 per

The Rockport Walking Test

In the test you will walk a mile then immediately count your heart rate (pulse rate). You will check the accompanying charts to find your fitness.

1. Find a flat, measured quarter-mile track, or measure a course. (You might drive your car a mile on a road then mark the 1 mile distance.)
2. Warm up by walking a few hundred yards at a leisurely pace.
3. With a stop watch, or a watch with a second hand, note the time you started.
4. Walk as fast as possible for an exact mile.
5. Note the time you took in minutes and seconds: _____ : _____
6. Immediately count your pulse rate for 15 seconds then multiply it by four to get your pulse per minute. You can put your finger on the opposite wrist, just above the thumb or feel the pulse in the side of your neck under the muscle about 2in (5cm) below your ear, or just put your hand over your heart.

(Number of heart beats for 15 seconds _____ × 4 = _____ pulse rate per minute.)

Finding Your General Fitness Level Through the Rockport Walking Test

7. Check the accompanying charts (Fig 12). Find the proper chart for your age and sex. Find the level of your heart rate (pulse) on the left side of the chart. Be exact. Draw a horizontal line from that point across the chart.
8. Find the amount of time it took you to walk the mile on the bottom of the chart. Find the closest spot within 10 seconds of your time. (Example – If you walked the mile in 14 minutes and 8 seconds, mark the spot about ⅛ of the way between the 14 and the 15 mark.) Draw a line directly upwards from that point.
9. The point where the two lines intersect will be in a light or dark area. Your general condition will be noted in that coloured area.

Measuring Your VO₂ Max Through the Rockport Fitness Walking Test

1. Your time for the mile walk (from number 5 above). _____ : _____
2. Convert the seconds to hundredths of a minute. (For instance, if your walk time was 10 minutes, 15 seconds = 10.25. This is the number you will put into the following formulas.
3. Use the following gender-specific formulae to determine maximal oxygen consumption rates (VO_2 max):

Male

_____ = 0.0947 × your body weight
_____ = 0.3709 × your age
_____ = 3.9744 × your mile time
_____ = 0.1847 × pulse rate after the mile
_____ (from number 6 in previous list.)
_____ *Total points*

Take 154.899 and subtract the above total to determine your VO_2 max.

154.899 – _____ – _____ Your VO_2 max
                (total points)

Female

_____ = 0.0585 × your body weight
_____ = 0.3885 × your age
_____ = 2.7961 × your mile time
            (in minutes and hundredths of a
            minute) (from number 2 above)
_____ = 0.1109 × mile heart rate pulse rate
            after the mile (from number 6 in
            previous list)
_____ *Total points*

Take 116.579 and subtract the above total to determine your VO_2 max.

116.579 – _____ = _____ Your VO_2 max

Fig 12. Finding your general fitness level.

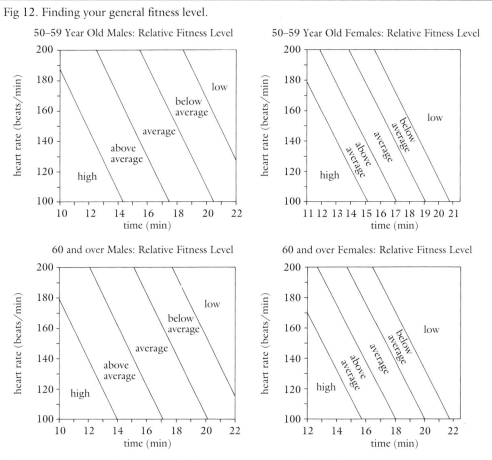

Low = Introductory level; Below average = Beginner; Average = Advanced beginner; Above average = Intermediate; High = High intermediate to advanced

Suggested Exercise Programme Based on Rockport One Mile Test

IF LOW TO BELOW AVERAGE FITNESS LEVEL

Week	1–2	3–4	5	6	7–8	9	10	11	12–13	14	15–16	17–18	19–20
Warm-up/ cool down*	5–7	5–7	5–7	5–7	5–7	5–7	5–7	5–7	5–7	5–7	5–7	5–7	5–7
Mileage	1.0	1.25	1.5	1.5	1.75	2.0	2.0	2.0	2.25	2.5	2.5	2.75	3.00
Pace (mph)	3.0	3.0	3.0	3.5	3.5	3.5	3.75	3.75	3.75	3.75	4.0	4.0	4.0
Heart rate (% of max)	60	60	60	60–70	60–70	60–70	60–70	70	70	70	70	70–80	70–80
Frequency (times per week)	5	5	5	5	5	5	5	5	5	5	5	5	5

*(stretches before and after walk in minutes)

continued overleaf

Suggested Exercise Programme Based on Rockport One Mile Test (continued)

IF BELOW AVERAGE TO AVERAGE

Week	1–2	3–4	5–6	7	8–9	10–12	13	14	15–16	17–18	19–20
Warm-up/ cool down*	5–7	5–7	5–7	5–7	5–7	5–7	5–7	5–7	5–7	5–7	5–7
Mileage	1.5	1.75	2.0	2.0	2.25	2.5	2.75	2.75	3.0	3.25	3.5
Pace (mph)	3.0	3.0	3.0	3.5	3.5	3.5	3.5	4.0	4.0	4.0	4.0
Heart rate (% of max)	60–70	60–70	60–70	70	70	70	70–80	70–80	70–80	70–80	70–80
Frequency (times per week)	5	5	5	5	5	5	5	5	5	5	5

IF AVERAGE TO ABOVE AVERAGE

Week	1	2	3–4	5	6–8	9–10	11–12	13–14	15	16–17	18–20	maintenance
Warm-up/ cool down*	5–7	5–7	5–7	5–7	5–7	5–7	5–7	5–7	5–7	5–7	5–7	5–7
Mileage	2	2.25	2.5	2.75	2.75	3.0	3.0	3.25	3.5	3.5	4.0	4.0
Pace (mph)	3.0	3.0	3.0	3.0	3.5	3.5	4.0	4.0	4.0	4.5	4.5	4.5
Heart rate (% of max)	70	70	70	70	70	70	70–80	70–80	70–80	70–80	70–80	
Frequency (times per week)	5	5	5	5	5	5	5	5	5	5	5	3–5

IF ABOVE AVERAGE TO HIGH

Week	1	2	3–4	5	6	7	8	9–10	11–14	15–20	maintenance
Warm-up/ cool down*	5–7	5–7	5–7	5–7	5–7	5–7	5–7	5–7	5–7	5–7	5–7
Mileage	2.5	2.75	3.0	3.25	3.5	3.5	3.75	4.0	4.0	4.0	4.0
Pace (mph)	3.5	3.5	3.5	3.5	3.5	4.0	4.0	4.0	4.5	4.5	4.5
Heart rate (% of max)	70	70	70	70	70–80	70–80	70–80	70–80	70–80	70–80	70–80
Frequency (times per week)	5	5	5	5	5	5	5	5	5	5	5

*(stretches before and after walk in minutes)

cent higher average VO_2 max than females. Age also influences it. A 20-year-old male will probably average 50, a 40-year-old will probably drop to 40, and a 70-year-old to 30. The top conditioned athlete in the world has a 95 VO_2 max. While you will never achieve to that 95 level of conditioning, you can certainly improve your own level through exercise. To determine your maximal oxygen consumption rate (VO_2 max), you can do the Rockport Fitness Walking Test[9], see p.116, as this has been validated by ACSM as an appropriate fitness test.

Now that you know your maximal oxygen consumption, you can test to see if your cardiorespiratory fitness programme is working by occasionally repeating the above test. As your fitness level increases, your VO_2 max will increase because cardiorespiratory fitness relies on the effective delivery and use of oxygen to make energy.

TO BEGIN A CARDIOVASCULAR FITNESS PROGRAMME

If you are in poor or average condition and desire to increase your fitness level, be sure that you begin with a low intensity activity such as walking or use a low intensity level on a stationary bike or a stair climber. Whichever approach you take, start slowly. If you begin any exercise programme too quickly, you will probably have some muscle soreness for the first few days. This soreness discourages some people, but it will disappear and will probably never return as you get into condition and keep fit. Any exercise-caused muscle soreness will peak in 2 days and be completely gone in 5 to 7 days. Keep improving by increasing the amount of time spent exercising and/or the intensity at which you exercise. Eventually, you will reach your fitness objectives, then you can continue to work at that level for maintenance.

Just about any time is a good time to exercise. However, if you exercise just before going to bed, you will increase your metabolism, which may make it more difficult to get to sleep. If you exercise just after eating, you will force your body to divide the available blood between the stomach, which needs it for digestion, and the skeletal muscles, which need it for exercise. But if you exercise just before a meal time you may find that you then don't desire as much food. If you use your exercise sessions to give you energy, you may choose to exercise in the morning. If you use your exercise sessions to relieve the stress and tension of your day, the evening would be a more appropriate time.

Warming Up and Cooling Down

Endurance exercise requires a proper warm-up, a vigorous activity period and a cool-down session. Even well-conditioned people often

---

Beginning Walking Programme

Week	Target Zone Exercising	Total Time (minutes) *
1	Walk briskly 5 min	15
2	Walk briskly 7 min	17
3	Walk briskly 9 min	19
4	Walk briskly 11 min	21
5	Walk briskly 13 min	23
6	Walk briskly 15 min	25
7	Walk briskly 18 min	28
8	Walk briskly 20 min	30
9	Walk briskly 23 min	33
10	Walk briskly 26 min	36
11	Walk briskly 28 min	38
12	Walk briskly 30 min	40

13 on: Check your pulse periodically to see if you are exercising within your target zone.

As you get more in shape, try exercising within the upper range of your target heart zone. Remember that your goal is to continue getting the benefits you seek while enjoying your activity.

* (warm-up + target zone exercising + cool-down)

Reproduced with permission. *Walking for a Healthy Heart*, American Heart Association.

---

show abnormal electrocardiograms when they exercise without a proper warm-up. However, they will show normal electrocardiograms when they are 'warmed up' prior to exercising. A warm-up is designed to increase blood flow to the muscles that you are going to work. So, a brisk walk would be an appropriate warm up to a jog, and a few minutes on a rowing machine or a slow swim would get the blood flowing to your upper body before a swimming workout. You can also perform the activity you plan to engage in for your workout at a very light intensity. A good indication that you are properly warmed up is when you begin to sweat. Five minutes is usually sufficient to get your body ready for your workout.

There are different reasons to stretch before or after a workout. If you want to increase your flexibility you would definitely want to stretch after your workout. However, stretching before a workout may set you up for injuries. Research is finding that runners tend to have more injuries if they stretch than if they don't, and swimmers don't swim as fast if they have stretched. Stretching cold muscles increases your chance of injury, so if you do want to stretch before you exercise it is better to do so after you have warmed up. If you are trying to increase your flexibility, you may choose to stretch after your cool-down, as your muscles are guaranteed to be warmed up after your intensive workout. In fact, stretching after exercise is more important than stretching before in terms of increasing your flexibility.

Cooling down after an exercise period is important if the exercise has been vigorous. It is suggested that the activity be slowed until the heart rate has reached a rate of about 100 beats per minute. When a person stops immediately after exercising, a great deal of blood may pool in the veins which may decrease the amount of blood available to the brain. If a person does not cool down properly, dizziness or fainting is possible – shock, and even a heart attack, are remote possibilities.

The best endurance exercises include cross country-skiing, running, swimming, aerobics, stair climbing, cycling, rowing as well as

---

Among the Types of Masters' Competition at the World Games

- Alpine skiing (slalom, giant slalom, Super G)
- Badminton (singles, doubles, mixed doubles)
- Basketball
- Biathlon
- Bowling (singles, doubles, team)
- Broomball
- Cross country skiing (30km men, 20km women, freestyle men 15km, 50km, women 10km and 30km)
- Curling
- Mixed curling
- Darts (singles, doubles, team)
- Diving
- Figure skating (ice dancing, precision skating),
- Handball (four-wall)
- Ice hockey
- Indoor archery
- Indoor athletics 50m to 5,000m, 10km, 50m hurdles, 1,500 and 5,000m walk, high jump, long jump, shot, triple jump, pentathlon
- Indoor shooting (pistol and rifle)
- Indoor football
- Indoor tennis (singles, doubles, mixed doubles)
- Judo
- Racquetball
- Ringette
- Snooker/billiards
- Speed skating (both short and long tracks)
- Squash
- Swimming
- Synchronized swimming
- Table tennis
- Team handball
- Triathlon
- Volleyball
- Water Polo (for men aged from 30)
- Weightlifting
- Wheelchair basketball
- Sledge hockey

General age group rule (some exceptions):

Men's groups (from 35): 35–39, 40–44, 45–49, 50–54, 55–59, and so on.
Women's groups (from 30): 30–34, 35–39, 40–44, and so on.
Disabled: 25 and up (one category).

walking on a treadmill or exercising on a bicycle exerciser. The least effective endurance exercises for cardiorespiratory fitness are weightlifting, callisthenics, archery and bowling as these are of no use in developing endurance.

Sports can be a vehicle to improving fitness. Handball, squash, tennis, football and basketball are vigorous enough to qualify as endurance exercise if played continuously for a long period of time. Most sports require some amount of athletic ability and many assist one in developing some amount of strength, flexibility and endurance. But the major benefit of most sports is that they allow us to relax while being active. Sports, especially the hitting sports such as tennis and badminton, or the body contact sports, such as football or basketball, can be great stress relievers. Of course, some people get 'uptight' about winning which may do more mental harm than good. If you like to compete, most countries now have 'Master' sports programmes which encourage participation or competition in your favourite sport.

MAKE IT FUN

Effective exercise is going to make you feel better physically and mentally. This will happen whether you enjoy the exercise or not. But why not enjoy it? If you enjoy swimming – swim. If you like to run – run. If you like to play golf – play. If you live in a country with cold winters you can do cross country skiing. If you like to dance – dance. It doesn't matter if it is ballet, country and western, swing or jazz, as long as your heart rate is increased. Anything that you do physically will help a little. Walk up the stairs at work. Take a walk while you talk at lunch.

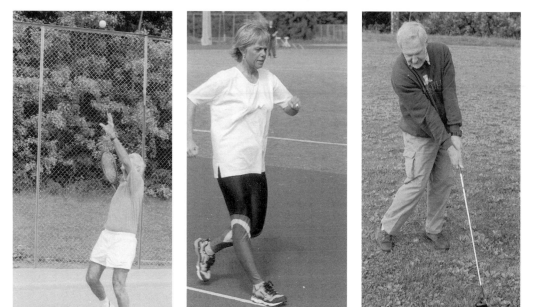

Fig 13. Tennis is enjoyed by many at every age.

Fig 14. Fitness walking is the simplest, least expensive and safest activity.

Fig 15. A five-mile walk along with the flexibility advantages of the sport make golf a preferred activity for many.

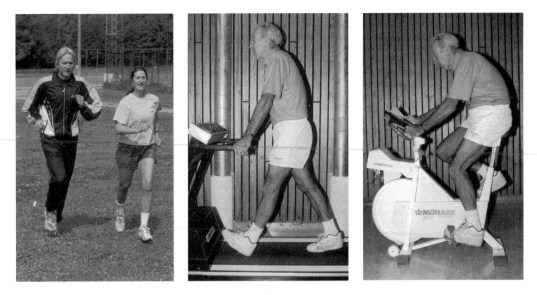

Fig 16. Jogging gives a highly effective workout in a shorter time than does walking.

Fig 17. Treadmill walking or running can be done at home or in a health club.

Fig 18. Cycling at home and catching up on reading.

If you like outdoor activities, run or walk your way to fitness. These are the most common approaches to exercise. Many of us like to walk the golf course for our exercise. A number of people are now enjoying orienteering. If you join an orienteering club, you will take your map and run from point to point as the map requires, so working your brain along with your legs. Orienteering is becoming increasingly popular, with national and international competitions.

Running, stair climbing or cycling may be boring for you. If so, you might try to make it entertaining by carrying a personal stereo with you while you jog. Or you might watch television or read while you exercise indoors on some form of stationary aerobic equipment. Try to do something to make exercise enjoyable for you, because the benefits you receive from it are well worth the effort!

Working out in a health studio environment is enjoyable for many people. You can lift weights with friends, ride the exercise bike in front of the television or watch a film, take an aerobics class, or take a 'spinning' class. In 'spinning' the class works out with an instructor. All are on exercise bikes. With the music, the instructor pedals forwards or backwards, fast or slow and the class mimics the instructor's movements.

Some of us like to work out at home because it doesn't involve any commuting time going to the gym. You can skip, follow an aerobics programme on television, or ride the exercise bike while watching television or reading. If you want to read you can buy a commercially made book holder which attaches to the bike's handlebars – or you can rummage around the local hardware store and make your own with plastic, clamps and tape.

If you are not already exercising effectively, are you motivated to look and feel better and to live longer? How strong is your motivation? You now have the knowledge necessary to begin an effective exercise programme.

Caloric Expenditure Chart

How many hours in the week did you use 480 calories (minimum for fitness; 750 calories is the recommended level for fitness)?

The following chart gives the various expenditures of calories for different types of activities which are expected during the exercise. Calories used per pound of body weight for 10 minutes of exercise.

(Cal./lb per 10 minutes)		
Activity		*10 min*
Archery		0.34
Baseball (except pitcher)		0.3
Callisthenics		0.34
Classwork, lecture		0.12
Cross-country running		0.8
Dancing (vigorously)		0.12
Downhill skiing		0.64
Dressing		0.2
Driving		0.2
Eating		0.09
Football (American)		0.54
Gardening, weeding		0.4
Golf		0.34
Housekeeping		0.6
Mountain climbing		0.67
Reading		0.06
Running:	7.0mph (11.3km/h)	0.93
	8.7mph (14km/h)	1.03
	11.6mph (18.7km/h)	1.31
Sitting		0.09
Sleeping		0.06

Soccer		0.6
Squash		0.7
Swimming:	pleasure	0.7
	breaststroke	0.64
	crawl 45yd	0.56
Table tennis		0.26
Tennis		0.46
Volleyball		0.26
Walking:	2.0mph (3.2km/h)	0.23
	4.5mph (7.2km/h)	0.44
Writing		0.09

To reach the 8 calories per minute level (80 calories per 10 minutes), multiply your weight by the number of calories used per pound (above). Does your exercise reach the 80 calories per 10-minute period? (If you do callisthenics at 0.34 calories per 10 minutes, you had better weigh 235lb (107kg) to get in your exercise. But if you swim you can get your minimum exercise if you weigh only 115lb (52kg)).

Remember to keep up your exercise for an hour if you are working only at the 80 calories per 10-minute level.

Has it changed your attitude? Will it change your behaviour?

When it comes to running for fun, Sir Roger Bannister may have said it best:

We run, not because we think it is doing us good, but because we enjoy it and cannot help ourselves. The more restricted our society and work become, the more necessary it will be to find some outlet for this craving for freedom. No one can say, 'You must not run faster than this, or jump higher than that.' The human spirit is indomitable.

Minimal fitness level by walking. It need not be continuous, but is cumulative throughout the day:

- Women – Walk 2 miles in under 30 minutes at least 3 days a week, or 2 miles in 30 to 40 minutes 6 or 7 days a week.
- Men – Walk 2 miles in under 27 minutes at least 3 days a week, or 2 miles in between 30 and 40 minutes 6 to 7 days per week.

(Steven Blair, Address at Pre-Olympic Scientific Congress, July 1992.)

CHAPTER 13
Strength Exercising for Muscles and Bones

National Institute on Aging, Gerontology Research Center, Baltimore, USA, has done a twenty-five year study on ageing men and women and the loss of strength and power (a combination of speed and strength). At about age 40 both strength and power declined in both sexes. However, power declined faster than strength in men.[1] With the loss of muscle cells and the reduction of physical work we can expect that strength will decrease. But many of us want to keep that loss minimal by exercising for strength and power.

The amount of strength one needs depends upon the type of occupation and recreational activities that are being performed. Both men and women need some strength. A female lorry driver needs more strength in her job than does a male secretary. She can gain the necessary strength by doing the proper exercises. But everyone needs some strength activity to keep the bones and muscles from becoming weaker – yes, the bones degenerate if they are not forced to support weight and osteoporosis can result.

There are four types of strength exercises:

- Concentric (isotonic) or dynamic exercises in which the muscle moves a joint through a certain range of motion, pushing the body upwards in a press-up or jumping up would be examples of concentric exercises;
- Isometric exercises in which the muscle contracts but does not move the joint – examples would be holding an object without moving it or standing in a doorway and pushing out on the door jamb;
- Eccentric contractions are those in which the muscle is lengthening rather than shortening during the exercise – an example would be lowering the body back to the floor during a press-up or landing on the ground after jumping upwards;
- Plyometric exercise is a combination of eccentric contractions quickly followed by concentric contractions – an example would be landing from a jump then rebounding into another jump.

Any one of these types of muscle contractions can aid you in gaining strength. However, the most commonly used is the concentric exercise. If you were trying to gain strength in your wrist to be able to serve a tennis ball better you would do a concentric exercise moving your wrist through a full range of motion.

There are two major factors which affect one's strength – the number of muscle fibres contracting at one time and the efficiency of the lever (joint and muscle attachments). A muscle is made up of thousands of small muscle fibres, each one about the size of a straight pin. Not all of the fibres in a muscle will contract at the same time, but every fibre contracting will do so to its maximum ability. This is known as the 'all or none' principle. The greater the percentage of fibres which a person can make contract at any one time, the greater the force which can be exerted.

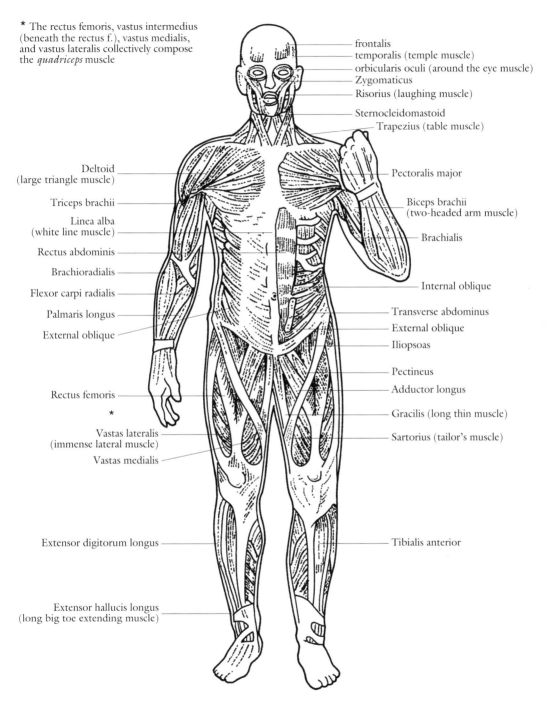

* The rectus femoris, vastus intermedius (beneath the rectus f.), vastus medialis, and vastus lateralis collectively compose the *quadriceps* muscle

frontalis
temporalis (temple muscle)
orbicularis oculi (around the eye muscle)
Zygomaticus
Risorius (laughing muscle)
Sternocleidomastoid
Trapezius (table muscle)

Deltoid (large triangle muscle)
Triceps brachii
Linea alba (white line muscle)
Rectus abdominis
Brachioradialis
Flexor carpi radialis
Palmaris longus
External oblique

Rectus femoris
*
Vastas lateralis (immense lateral muscle)
Vastas medialis

Extensor digitorum longus

Extensor hallucis longus (long big toe extending muscle)

Pectoralis major
Biceps brachii (two-headed arm muscle)
Brachialis
Internal oblique
Transverse abdominus
External oblique
Iliopsoas
Pectineus
Adductor longus
Gracilis (long thin muscle)
Sartorius (tailor's muscle)
Tibialis anterior

Fig 19. Muscles of the body, front view.

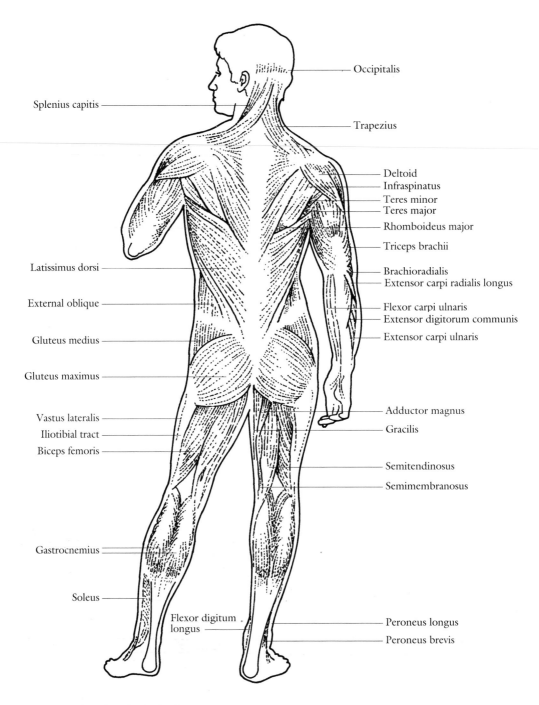

Occipitalis

Splenius capitis

Trapezius

Deltoid
Infraspinatus
Teres minor
Teres major
Rhomboideus major
Triceps brachii

Brachioradialis
Extensor carpi radialis longus

Latissimus dorsi

Flexor carpi ulnaris
Extensor digitorum communis

External oblique

Extensor carpi ulnaris

Gluteus medius

Gluteus maximus

Adductor magnus
Gracilis

Vastus lateralis
Iliotibial tract
Biceps femoris

Semitendinosus

Semimembranosus

Gastrocnemius

Soleus

Flexor digitum longus

Peroneus longus
Peroneus brevis

Fig 20. Muscles of the body, back view.

Every joint is a lever which varies in efficiency. The biceps muscle in the front of the upper arm works on a more efficient lever than does the calf muscle (gastrocnemius), which allows one to rise up on the toes. And levers also vary in efficiency from person to person. Those who have shorter bones generally have better lever actions than those with longer bones. Heavily muscled people generally have more efficient levers, as well as more muscle fibres, than do tall, thin people. This is why you don't see tall, thin competitors in Olympic weightlifting events.

While the ideal method of gaining strength is by the use of heavy resistance apparatus, such as is provided by barbells and dumbbells, it is possible to gain strength by using one's body as the resistance for the muscles. The following exercises do not require apparatus:

1. For the front of the chest (upper pectorals) and the back of the upper arms (triceps), do press-ups. If you cannot do a

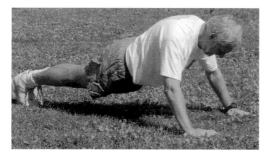

Fig 21. Standard press-up – for chest and triceps.

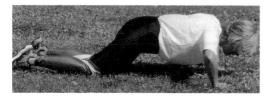

Fig 22. Modified press-up for those not strong enough for the standard press-up or for those seeking muscular endurance in the chest and triceps.

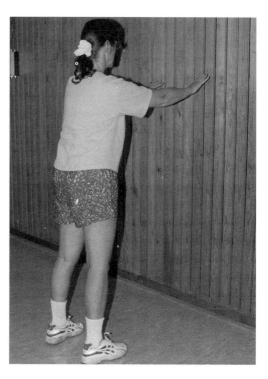

Fig 23. Wall pushaway. The simplest chest and triceps exercise.

regular press-up, the resistance can be reduced by keeping your knees on the floor or by pushing away from a wall.

2. For the front of the upper arms (biceps), lie on the floor. Bend your legs while

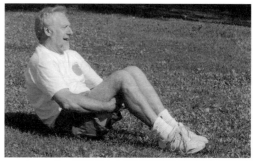

Fig 24. A simple biceps exercise – pull your chest up to your knees using your arms.

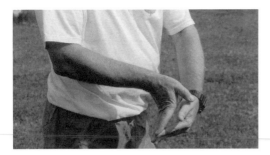

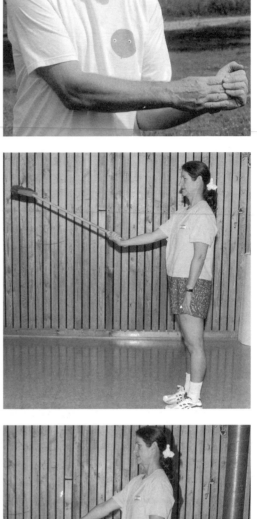

Fig 25. Manual resistance for increasing forearm strength.

Fig 26. Manual resistance for the back of the forearm – give resistance to the back of the fingers of the right arm while pulling the right hand backwards *(above, right)*.

Fig 27. Lifting a broom for forearm strength *(right)*.

Fig 28. Completing the broom lift *(below)*.

Fig 29. Broom lift for the back of the forearm *(below, right)*.

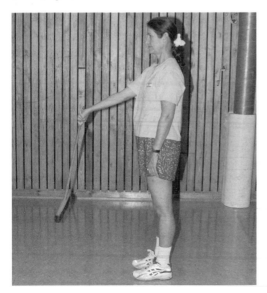

keeping your feet flat on the floor, lock your hands behind your thigh, and pull your head and shoulders up to the knees. This exercise will also stretch the back muscles. Another exercise for the biceps is to use your other hand to give you resistance while you bend your arm.

3. For the forearms, squeeze a tennis ball or push one hand against the other. You can also lift a broom with your wrist. As you become stronger, move your grip farther from the bristles of the broom – or get a heavier broom. Who knows, you might even work up to lifting a shovel! This broom exercise is particularly good for strengthening the wrist for a tennis serve if you hold the broom palm up and for the golf swing if it is held palm down.

4. For the neck, put your hand on your head (the front, back or side, depending on which muscles you wish to strengthen). Push the head against the hand. With pressure on the back of the head it will help to correct the postural defect of a 'forward head'.

5. For the upper leg, steady yourself by holding on to a table. Do a one-legged half-knee bend. Do not let the upper leg go past the position at which it is parallel to the floor. Connective tissue in the knee may be damaged if you do a full knee bend. If you are not strong enough to do a one-legged knee bend, do the exercise with both legs. By doing the exercise with one leg rather than two, you double the amount of weight which the leg muscles are forced to lift. This is good for skiing and running.

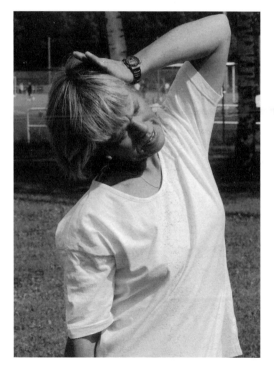

Fig 30. Side of neck exercise.

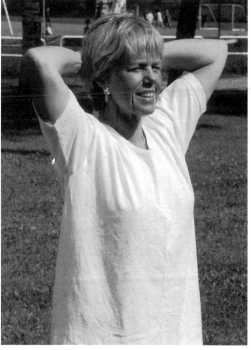

Fig 31. Back of the neck exercise – very important for posture.

129

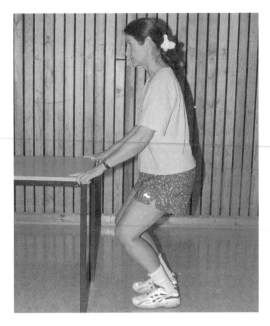

Fig 32. Half-knee bend using a table for balance.

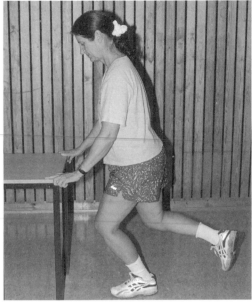

Fig 33. One leg half-knee bend – doubles the resistance of the two-leg knee bend.

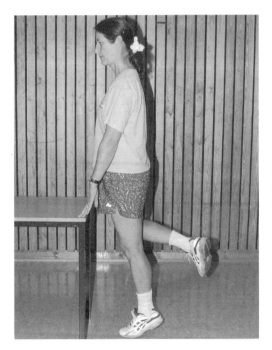

Fig 34. Single-leg calf exercise.

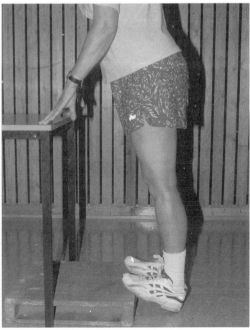

Fig 35. To increase the flexibility of the ankle.

6. For the lower leg, steady yourself by holding on to a table, then rise up on your toes. Do this one leg at a time. To get more stretch put the balls of your feet on a one to two inch block of wood then lower your heels to the floor. This is good for running. To get more stretch, stand on a block of wood.
7. Lifting any weight over your head will also put some stress on the vertebrae of your spine and help to prevent osteoporosis.

If you can do the exercises more than ten times, you need more resistance if they are to be the most effective strength exercises.

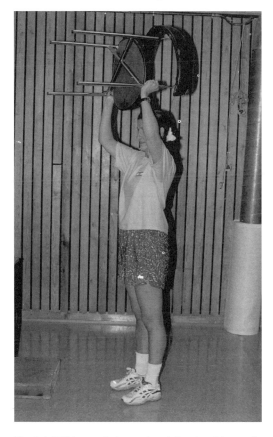

Fig 36. Lifting a chair overhead for shoulder and triceps strength.

RESISTANCE TRAINING FOR STRENGTH

The most common exercises done in gyms generally involve at least two muscle groups acting at the same time. For example, the bench press and the press-up both use the upper chest muscles and the back of the upper arms. It is impossible to determine just how much each muscle group is working when these exercises are done. For example, compare two people doing press-ups: one may be doing 55 per cent of the work with the chest muscles and 45 per cent with the triceps (the muscles in the back of the upper arm), while the other may be doing far more of the pushing with the triceps than the chest muscles.

For general strength conditioning, the exercises which use two muscle groups are fine. However, if you are a person who wants to develop each muscle to its greatest strength, it would be best to isolate the muscles you desire to develop. Competitive athletes are the people most likely to desire such optimum strength development. However, if you were a skier you might well concentrate on the muscles in the front of your thighs because they often tire first. A golfer might want to concentrate on wrist or abdominal strength.

There are two criteria for finding the best exercise for any muscle. First, the muscle group for which strength is to be developed should be isolated. Second, the joint involved should be exercised through the greatest range of motion possible. By doing this, the muscle and the connective tissue associated with that muscle will be stretched to the maximum. This gives the person maximum flexibility for that joint while still achieving maximum strength.

Another factor that is important in determining the greatest development of strength is that the muscle should be exercised until it is exhausted. This exhaustion should occur at about eight repetitions of the exercise. If you can do ten repetitions, the weight is too light for maximum strength development. However, if you don't need maximum strength just do what repetitions you can manage. Anything helps.

DO SAFE EXERCISES

Since there are some exercises which may damage tissue, they should be avoided. The previously mentioned deep knee bend or 'squat' is one. If a person does a full deep knee bend, the ligaments in the front of the knee begin to be stretched after the leg has been bent more than 90 degrees. If the knee bend is continued to the point where the calf muscles and the muscles at the back of the thigh touch, the stretching of the knee ligaments is greatly increased. So while a deep knee bend would strengthen the muscles which work the knee, it would weaken the internal structure of the knee joint. For most people this may not be a great problem, but for those who play golf, tennis or who ski, it can make the knee more susceptible to being sprained.

Any potentially harmful exercise which stretches the connective tissue in the abdominal area by bending too far back should be avoided. It is desirable to have tight connective tissue in the abdominal area to assist the muscles in supporting the visceral organs in the abdomen.

Another dangerous exercise is one that puts great pressure on the discs of the lower spine. The 'dead lift', in which one bends at the waist and lifts a heavy weight with the lower back muscles, is such an exercise. This exercise can put as much as 3,000 to 5,000lb of pressure per square inch on the lower spinal discs. Such pressure has ruptured the discs of some weight-lifters. It can also weaken the discs and make them more susceptible to injury later in life.

Pulling forwards on the neck, which was common in the older style of sit-ups, is also contra-indicated because it may stretch the connective tissues in the back of the cervical vertebrae.

The exercises which adhere to the above criteria – isolation of the muscle, maximum flexibility of the joint, and little chance of damage to the body – are illustrated on the weightlifting photos. Remember that as soon as you can do ten repetitions, you can add more weight for your next workout. Remember too that at age 50 you will have lost some muscle fibre so will not have the same potential for strength as you had at 20.

DESIGNING YOUR WEIGHT-TRAINING PROGRAMME

You must first decide what it is that you want. Do you want to lose weight, to increase your muscle size, to get stronger, to become more aerobically fit, to rehabilitate a muscle after an accident or surgery, or to become better at a particular sport? If you want more strength, power or larger muscles you would want to train with weights or other types of resistance.

Repetitions

The number of repetitions is important.

For *strength* use a heavy weight which you can lift for only one to three repetitions before your muscles are exhausted. Repeat this several times during your workout. This type of workout may affect the brain more than the muscles – teaching the brain to be able to contract a greater percentage of muscle fibres, thereby increasing one's strength. Most of us at 50 plus don't need maximum strength, but for those competing in Master's level competition it may still be desirable.

- For *hypertrophy* (bigger muscles) exhaust your muscles in sets of ten to twenty-five repetitions doing a total of 150 to 250 repetitions of the exercise during the workout. The continued repetitions increase the blood flow, increase the size of the connective tissue (tendons and tissues which hold the fibres together), as well as increasing the cross-sectional size of the individual muscle fibres. Recent research also indicates that more muscle fibres may be developed. It was once thought that a person could not increase the number of fibres in a muscle.

- For *muscle endurance* use a very light weight and do the exercise one hundred or more times. This brings more blood flow to the muscles and increases the number of slow twitch muscle fibres which can be utilized. Generally, it is better to perform the activity for which you want the endurance, such as swimming, cycling or running.

Effective Breathing

Breathing effectively while exercising is important in order to minimize the chance of hernia or of rupturing blood vessels while lifting heavy weights. The best method of breathing is to exhale while lifting the weight. The second best method is to inhale while lifting. Holding the breath is the most dangerous because the air pressure inside the chest cavity is increased when the muscles around the ribs and shoulders are contracting. This is called the Valsalva manoeuvre or Valsalva effect. The strain of the increased internal air pressure can push part of the intestine through the inguinal rings (holes) of the lower hip bone, causing an inguinal hernia.

DEVELOPING MUSCULAR ENDURANCE

It is not enough to have your heart healthy and more red blood cells. Your individual muscles also have to have specific endurance. The muscles you use in an endurance activity will develop a better capacity to use the oxygen and sugars which the blood brings to them. There will be more haemoglobin in the muscles, more readily available fuel, and there may even be a different type of muscle tissue developed.

There are three different types of muscle fibres, the slow twitch (red or type I), the intermediate (type IIa), and the fast twitch (white or type IIb). The fast twitch fibres contract quickly but cannot do this for many repetitions. Olympic weightlifters have a high percentage of these because they need only one powerful contraction, then they rest for many minutes. Endurance athletes, such as cross-country skiers, swimmers and distance runners have a large percentage of the slow twitch fibres. These fibres contain more fuel and can contract many times. Alpine skiers are somewhere in-between.

Research indicates that the type of training a person does can change the type of fibres present. It may be that the intermediate fibres which change more towards the fast or slow twitch type of fibre.

INCREASING YOUR STRENGTH

Muscular endurance and muscular strength are at opposite ends of the spectrum. Strength is how much force you can generate in one muscular contraction while endurance is how long you can continue muscular contractions with relatively little resistance against them. If you are a skier, you will never require an absolute maximum force such as an Olympic weightlifter would need, but there are times when you will need more than the normal amount of power. Your extra strength will even help you to get up after a fall, so more strength will be necessary at times. And when running or walking up a hill more than the average amount of strength will be needed for a number of muscular contractions.

Your strength is determined primarily by the number of individual muscle fibres you can have contracting in one contraction. No one can contract all of the muscle fibres in a muscle at the same time; few people can even contract 50 per cent at one time. So your strength training programme is designed to teach your brain to be able to contract more muscle fibres at one time.

The following exercises will help you to condition your muscles. If you are trying to get stronger, exhaust your muscles in under ten repetitions. Exhaustion in one to three repetitions is best. But if you are working on developing muscular endurance, such as you will need during a long run, do a number of repetitions. You will be able to tell whether your are developing your muscular endurance by how your 'quads' feel at the end of the day.

A good range for most people would be twenty-five to one hundred. But remember that your muscles should be exhausted when you finish. It is only by getting your muscles very tired that you will achieve the best results. However, remember that anything is better than nothing.

The following strength exercises will help to condition you for skiing in particular:

The Abdominal Curl-Up

The abdominals are important for posture, for running and any running sport, walking and skiing. Everyone knows this exercise but some have not kept up with the latest techniques to make it more effective. Lie on the floor, or on your bed:

- put your hands on your chest (to avoid pulling in on the neck muscles);
- bring your feet up as close to your hips as

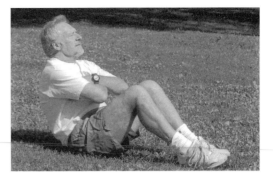

Fig 37. Abdominal curl-up (keep belt on the ground and look upwards).

possible (so that you don't use the small hip flexing muscles which attach to the lower back – especially important for women);
- look at the ceiling and continue looking at the same spot during the exercise (so that you don't stretch the muscles in the back of your neck); then
- raise your shoulders and concentrate on bringing the lower part of your ribs closer to the top of your hips;
- do as many repetitions as you can because you want muscular endurance from these muscles.

There are actually four sets of muscles in the abdominal wall. One, the rectus abdominis, does most of the work in the sit-up. There are two sets of angled muscles called the 'obliques'. These also assist in the sit-up as well as in the twisting and sideward-bending actions. The following exercises work on the 'obliques.'

The Twisting Abdominal Curl-Up

This exercise is done in the same way as the above exercise, but as you raise your shoulders you bring your right shoulder towards your left knee on one repetition, then your left shoulder to your right knee on the next one.

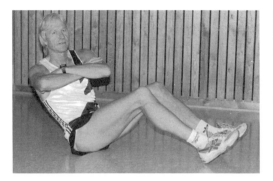

Fig 38. Twisting sit-up for the side abdominal (oblique) muscles.

Fig 39. Rotary abdominal machine *(right)*.

Fig 40. Side sit-ups for abdominal and lower back muscles on the lifting side.

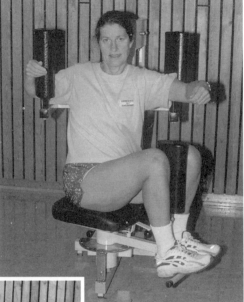

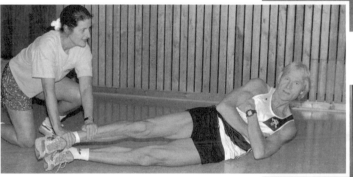

Fig 41. Lying leg rotation for abdominal muscles *(below)*.

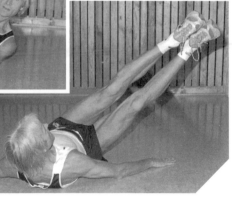

If you belong to a gym there may be a rotary abdominal machine – if so, it is more effective than the twisting sit-up.

Another exercise which can develop the abdominal obliques is the side sit-up. Put your feet under a sofa or have someone hold them down, then, while on your side, bring your shoulders and torso upwards.

Another particularly good exercise is done lying on the floor on your back. Extend your legs straight over your hips. With your arms out to your side to keep your torso flat, allow your legs to come down to the right side, then bring them back up, then down to the left side.

Shoulder Extension

This is another important exercise for most people to do unless they have been swimmers or gymnasts. The upper back and back of the arm muscles are not used often, but it is an important area to prevent osteoporosis in the upper back.

If you belong to a gym, use a pull-down pulley and pull it down with your arms straight. If you don't belong to a gym, you can buy stretching bands at a sporting goods shop or surgical tubing (about 8 to 10ft/2.4 to 2.5m) from a pharmacy. Screw an eye bolt into a door jamb or into a wall in the garage, and anchor the middle of the band to the bolt. Tie knots in the end of the tubes, or make a handle, then pull – alternating arms or using both arms together.

The Triceps

The triceps (three heads) straighten (extend) the elbow. One of the three heads crosses the shoulder joint so it works with the 'lats' in pulling the upper arm backwards. All three heads work to straighten the arm at the elbow joint.

If you belong to a gym, use the triceps extension machine or do triceps extensions on the 'lat' pull-down machine. You can also raise a dumbbell over your head. If you don't

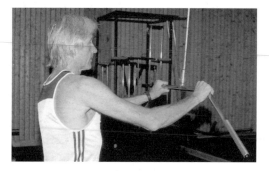

Fig 42. Pull down on the 'lat' machine for upper back and rear of shoulders.

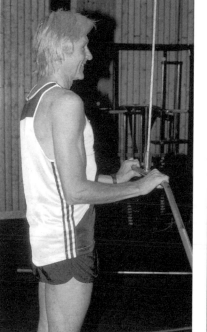

Fig 43. Tricep exercise on 'lat' machine (the elbows remain at the side of the body during the exercise – only the elbow joint moves).

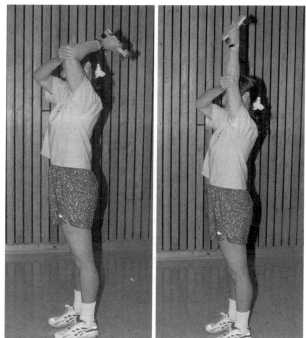

Fig 44. Triceps exercise holding a dumbell (a book will do). Hold the elbow next to the ear with the non-exercising hand.

Fig 45. Finish of triceps exercise *(right)*.

belong to a gym, you can do press-ups with either your feet or your knees on the floor.

The Biceps

These are used whenever you flex your arm. Take dumbbells, books, or bricks and lift.

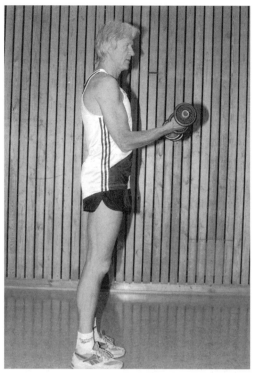

Fig 47. Biceps curl using a dumbell (book, brick, bucket of water, and so on).

The Front of the Thigh

The front of the thigh, or quadriceps, helps you to run, walk, ski or cycle. It holds your leg in that bent leg position which is critical to down-hill skiing. There is no question that these are the most important muscles for the alpine skier. You will want both muscular strength and muscular endurance in this group.

If you are in a gym, use the quadriceps machine. If not, get a partner. Sit on a table. Have your partner place both hands on your

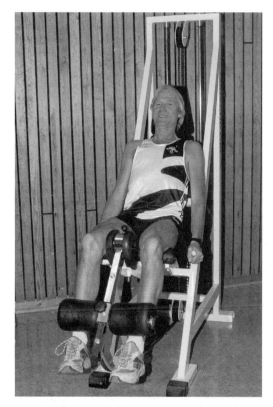

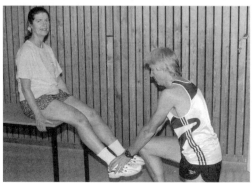

Fig 46. Quadriceps (front of thigh) exercise on quadriceps machine (*above left*).

Fig 48. Qaudriceps exercise using a partner for resistance (*left*).

ankle to provide resistance. You straighten your leg. If you don't have a partner, you can use that same rubber band as was recommended for the upper back.

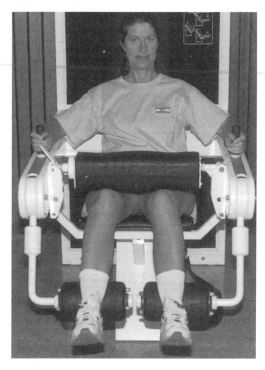

Fig 49. Hamstring (back of thigh) exercise on one type of hamstring machine.

Fig 50. Hamstring exercise with partner providing resistance to back of heel.

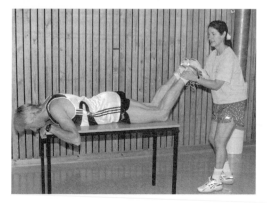

The Back of the Thigh

The back of the thigh, or hamstrings, must be strong to counterbalance the quadriceps. Gyms have special machines for the hamstrings. If you don't have access to one, get your trusty old partner, lie face down on the floor or a table, and have your partner push against your ankle as you lift your lower leg from the floor. Keep the other knee on the floor.

The Back of the Hips

The back of the hips, or gluteals, work in any walking, running, cycling or skiing action. They are also critical for posture. To work the upper part of the rear of the hips, the muscles that do a lot of your power work, with your quads, lie on a table face down with your hips on the table but your thighs past the table and your toes touching the floor. You can use a partner, if you want more strength, or do it alone, if you want more endurance by doing many repetitions. Start with one toe touching the floor while the other leg is brought as high as possible, then alternate legs. This will look like an exaggerated kicking action for a person swimming the crawl stroke.

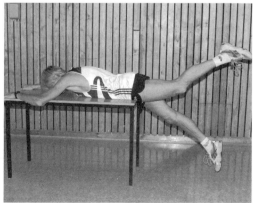

Fig 51. Buttock and hamstring exercise on table.

Hip and Knee Extension

This gives you greater force potential from your hips and knees. Gyms all have either squat racks, sleds or other machines which allow you to extend your legs. However, this exercise can be done easily at home. You can just do a three-quarter (*see* Figs 32 & 33) knee bend (don't bend your knees more than 90 degrees) or you can do half-knee bends. If you want twice the amount of resistance, do your knee bends with only one leg. To do a half knee bend, hold a table top to steady yourself. Using only one leg bend down 45 to 90 degrees then return to a standing position. By doing it on only one leg, you get the same effect as doing it with two legs while holding a barbell equal to your own weight.

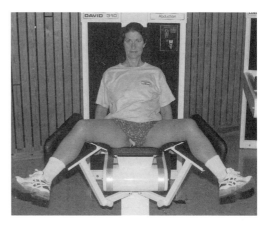

Fig 52. Hip abduction (thighs moving outwards) on machine.

Calf Muscles

The calf muscles, or gastrocnemius, are exercised by simply rising up on your toes then bringing your heels back to the ground. Repeat many times for endurance. If you want more strength, such as for hill climbing, balance yourself by holding a table or chair, then do the exercise using only one leg at a time, until each one is exhausted (*see* Figs 34 & 35).

Hip Abductors

The hip abductors move your legs sideways away from the mid-line of your body. They are very important in helping you to maintain your balance.

Some gyms have special machines for the abductors. If there is a 'multi-hip' machine, use it. Most gyms have low pulley weights with ankle straps. Stand with one side of your body next to the machine and put the ankle strap on the leg farthest from the machine. Lift the leg sideways keeping it straight.

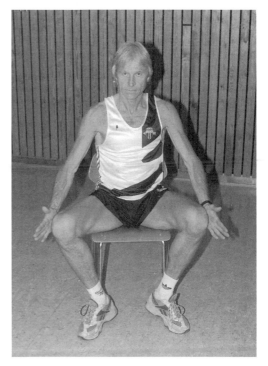

Fig 53. Manual resistance for hip abduction.

With a partner, lie on your side. Let your partner put pressure on your knee or ankle,

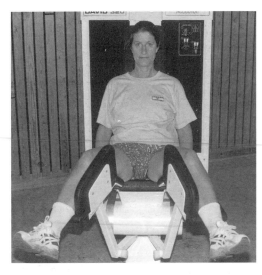

Fig 54. Hip adduction (thighs moving in) on machine.

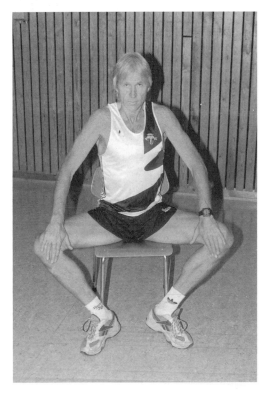

Fig 55. Hip adduction with manual resistance.

then lift your leg as high as you can. If you have no partner, you can do the same exercise alone – you just won't get as strong, but you can achieve just as much endurance.

You can also use the rubber bands. Attach one to a low part of a wall, hook your foot into a loop on the end of the band, and lift your leg outwards.

Hip Adductors

These muscles are high on the inside of your thighs. They also help in balancing. In addition, they bring your legs back together if they have been moved outward by the abductors. The exercises are the reverse of those for the abductors.

If your gym has a machine, use it. If there is a low pulley station, stand sideways to the pulley, but a yard away from the machine. Put the ankle strap on the ankle nearest the machine. Let your leg move outwards (towards the machine) with the weight, then bring it back to the other leg.

With a partner, lie on your back. Spread your legs. Let your partner give pressure inside your ankles. Bring your legs back together. If you wish, you can combine the adductor and abductor muscles in this exercise. As you lie on your back, your partner will provide hand pressure on the outside of both ankles. You will spread your legs against the pressure (abductors). Then your partner will provide pressure on the inside of your ankles and you will bring your legs back together (adductors).

Without a partner, just sit on the floor or on a chair with your feet about 12in (30cm) from your hips, with the heels together. Spread your knees outwards, then grasp the inside of your knees with your hands. Bring your knees together as you resist the movement with your hands. You will feel the tension inside your upper thighs.

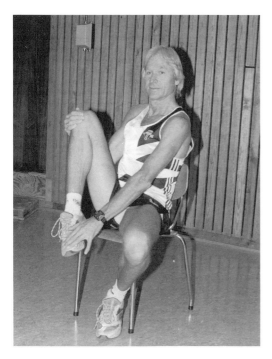

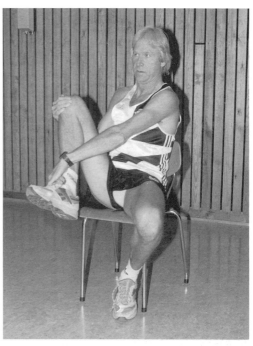

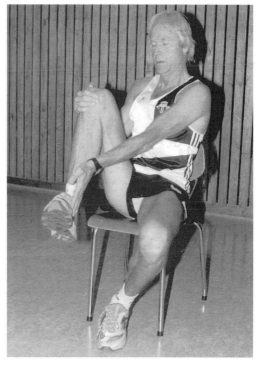

Fig 56. Ankle dorsi-flexion (toes moving towards shin). Very useful for walkers and runners *(above)*.

Fig 57. Outside of ankle exercise *(above right)*.

Fig 58. Inside of ankle exercise. Very useful for walkers and runners *(right)*.

Inside and Outside Calf Muscles

The muscles inside and outside of your calf also aid in balance. They should be strong enough to bring you back easily to a balanced position. The best way to work these muscles is to sit down, cross one leg over the other with your raised foot just past your other knee. Place one hand on the outside of the foot and move your foot outwards as you resist with your hand. (The scientific name for this movement is 'eversion.') Then put the other hand on the inside of the foot, near the ball of your foot, and resist as you bring your foot inwards (inversion).

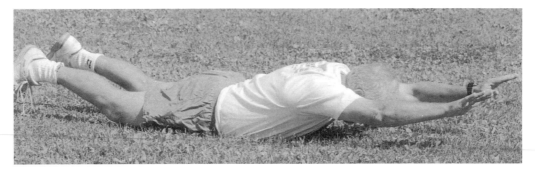

Fig 59. Slight back extension for lower back.

Lower Back

Exercises for the lower back should be more geared towards muscular endurance than strength, so you will want many repetitions. For most people, it is the most important exercise to do because there are so many lower back problems related to muscular weakness. You can lie on the floor face down and lift your shoulders about 6in (15cm) from the floor, then return to the floor. (Avoid going too high with your shoulders as you don't want to create a 'sway back' in your exercise.

You can also do this with a partner. With the partner holding your legs, and your hips and legs on a table, bend forwards at the waist to 60 or 90 degrees then lift your torso back up so that it is in line with your legs and hips. Again, you don't want to arch your back during the exercise.

How Many Repetitions and How Much Weight?

How many repetitions you do and how much weight you use depends on your goals. For pure strength, the muscle should be exhausted in one to three repetitions. However, pure strength is not what you want for skiing. You want a certain amount of strength and you want muscular endurance. So you will want from twenty to over one hundred repetitions. Of course, anything you do will help.

With a partner, using your own 'manual resistance' can actually be better than using weights. Your partner can adjust the pressure to make you work to a maximum level on each repetition. Weights cannot do this. Only partners and 'isokinetic' machines have this capability. So if you are using a partner don't think that you're not getting the best strength workout. In fact that partner is probably entitled to a good dinner once a week for helping you to develop your 'habit.'

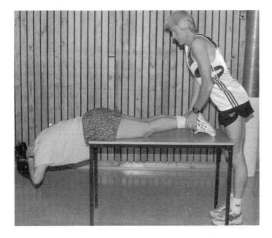

Fig 60. Back extension on table.

CHAPTER 14
Flexibility and Posture

Flexibility results when a person stretches connective tissue: ligaments (which hold bone to bone); tendons (which hold muscle to bone); fascia (a sheet of connective tissue); and small pieces of connective tissue which hold the muscle fibres together. On the muscle chart on page 125–6, the connective tissue appears in white.

Connective tissue shrinks somewhat if it is not stretched often. We frequently feel a tightness in the lower back or a lessened ability to touch our toes as we age. However, shrunken or tightened connective tissue can be stretched relatively easily, and normal flexibility can usually be regained within a few weeks, if the proper stretching exercises are done daily. It is never too late to start. A recent study of women with an average age of 72 showed significant increases in flexibility after a 10-week stretching programme.[1] We actually need more stretching as we age because of the tightness and the loss of elasticity in our muscle fibres.

One of the chief causes of poor posture is tight connective tissue. When the tissue in the front of the shoulders is allowed to shrink, it pulls the shoulders forwards resulting in round shoulders. When the tissue connecting the lower hips to the thigh is allowed to shorten, it pulls the hips forwards and a 'pot belly' develops. Pot belly can also be caused by too much beer, too many cakes, and weak abdominal muscles.

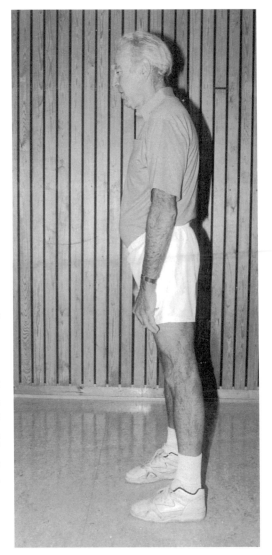

Fig 61. Poor posture (pot belly, forward shoulders, forward head).

Fig 62. The skeletal structure of the body, front view.

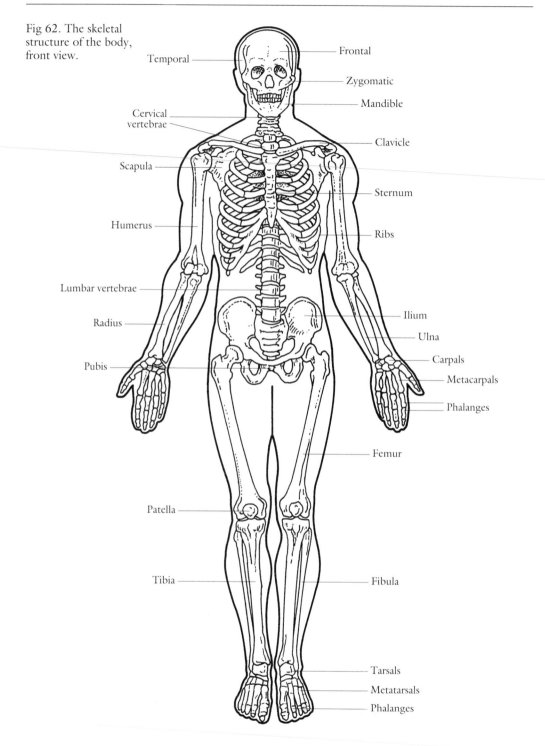

Temporal

Frontal

Zygomatic

Mandible

Cervical vertebrae

Clavicle

Scapula

Sternum

Humerus

Ribs

Lumbar vertebrae

Ilium

Radius

Ulna

Carpals

Pubis

Metacarpals

Phalanges

Femur

Patella

Tibia

Fibula

Tarsals

Metatarsals

Phalanges

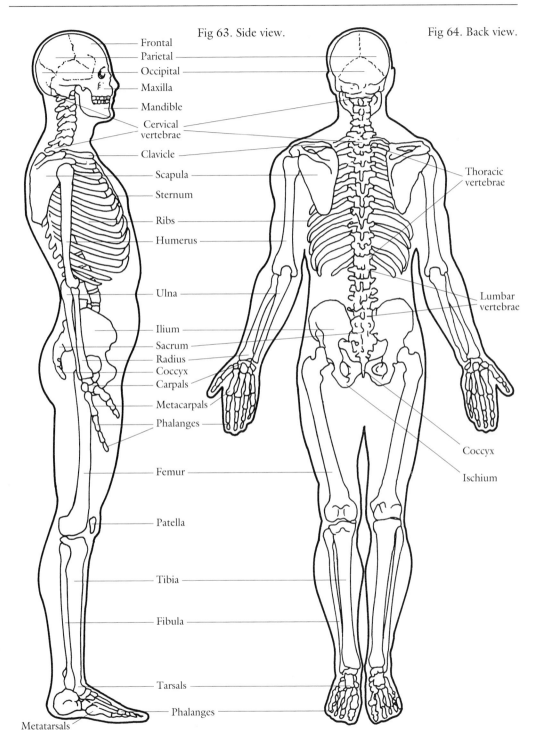

Fig 63. Side view.

Fig 64. Back view.

Frontal
Parietal
Occipital
Maxilla
Mandible
Cervical vertebrae
Clavicle
Scapula
Sternum
Ribs
Humerus
Ulna
Ilium
Sacrum
Radius
Coccyx
Carpals
Metacarpals
Phalanges
Femur
Patella
Tibia
Fibula
Tarsals
Phalanges
Metatarsals

Thoracic vertebrae
Lumbar vertebrae
Coccyx
Ischium

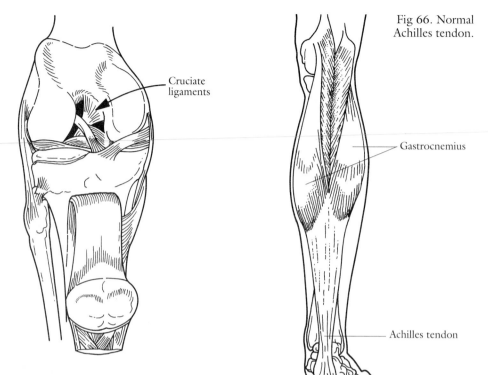

Cruciate
ligaments

Fig 66. Normal
Achilles tendon.

Gastrocnemius

Achilles tendon

Fig 65. Front view of knee.

Two flexibility exercises which help to prevent poor posture (or assist in regaining good posture) are the chest stretcher and the lower hip stretcher.

The exercise which best stretches the front of the shoulders is done by pulling the shoulders and arms back as far as they can go in a slow stretch. This not only stretches the front of the shoulder area, but also strengthens the upper back which will aid in helping to pull the shoulders back.

The exercise which best stretches the front of the lower hip area is done by taking a normal stride forwards, tightening the abdominal muscles (so that they will not be stretched) then pushing the hips forwards until the stretch is felt in the front of the lower hips.

Three exercises for general flexibility should also be done. The best exercise for trunk flexibility involves twisting the body as far as it will go. Push with the shoulder to accentuate the twisting action. The stretch is very good for the lower back and may be felt in the knees or ankles, if done correctly.

The best exercise for stretching the lower back and the back of the thighs is carried out in a sitting position. Reach down as far as possible. This exercise is more effective when sitting than when standing because the back of the thighs are relaxed when sitting. When standing they are under tension.

Stretching the calf muscle (back of the lower leg) is done by standing a few feet from a wall, placing the hands on the wall, and with the

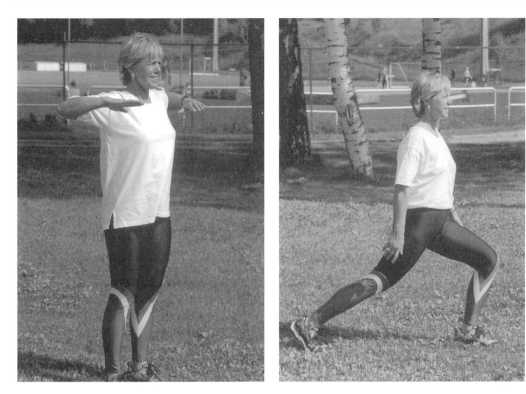

Fig 67. Upper back exercise to reduce forward shoulder slouch.

Fig 68. Front of hip stretch to reduce pot belly. Tighten the abdominal muscles and feel the stretch in the front of the hip.

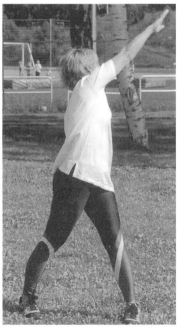

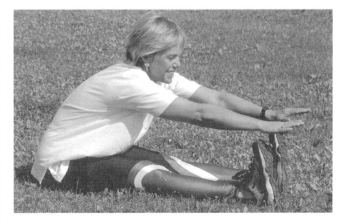

Fig 69. Trunk twist *(left)*.

Fig 70. Lower back and hamstring stretch *(above)*.

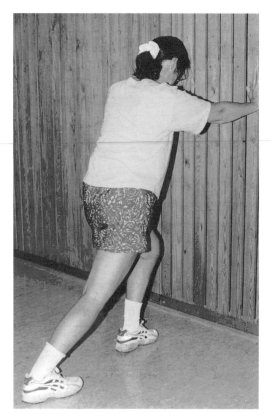

Fig 71. Calf stretch against a wall.

feet flat on the floor lean forwards from the ankles until you feel the stretch in the calf muscle and heel cord (Achilles tendon). Women who have worn high heel shoes generally have allowed the Achilles tendon to shorten more than normal so will need additional stretching.

GOOD POSTURE

Good posture requires not only the flexibility to allow the shoulders and hips to be able to assume the proper alignment, but also the strength to hold that alignment. The major muscle groups which hold one in a good posture are: the gluteal muscles of the buttocks, which pull down on the back of the hips, in turn raising the front of the hips; the abdominal muscles, which pull up on the front of the hips; the lower back muscles, which pull down on the rib cage, raising the chest; and the upper back muscles which hold the shoulders back.

The best exercise for the abdominal muscles is the curl-up. While sitting on the floor with the knees bent, the trunk is curled forwards as far as possible without letting the belt (top of hips) rise from the floor. Keeping the hips on the floor and the knees bent makes it nearly impossible to use the muscles in the lower hip area. These are the muscles which tend to pull the hips forwards, giving one a pot belly and a sway back. Put your hands on your chest, look up at the ceiling, and curl forwards. This exercise should be done between ten to fifty times each day. If you can't do the exercise, grab the back of your thighs with your hands and pull yourself up. In this way your biceps will aid you in doing the curl-up.

If you are not sufficiently strong to perform the abdominal curl-up, there is a progression of exercises which can be done to strengthen the muscles. Lie on the floor. If you are very weak, bend one leg then lift it towards your shoulders. (Very few people are so weak that they have to start with this exercise.) The next level of progression is lifting both legs bent. When you can do this ten times you will be ready for the real curl-up – holding the back of the thighs.

The exercise which strengthens all of the back muscles is the back extension. Raise the shoulders and legs upwards 2 to 4in (5 to 10cm), then relax. This should also be done ten to fifty times. This may be the most important exercise one can do, since the lower back muscles are the most often injured. We must therefore keep them as strong as possible to minimize the chance of injury. Lower back pain afflicts nearly seven million people. It is often a result of poor posture, but can be

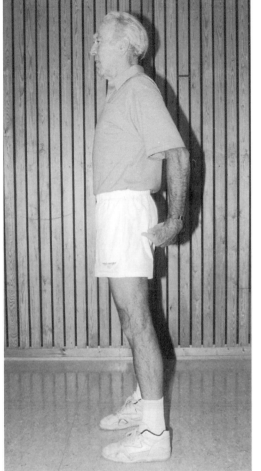

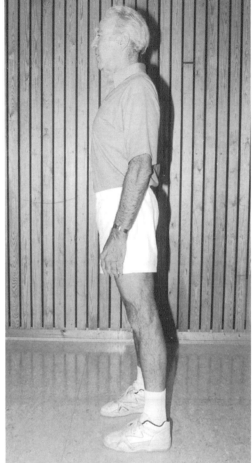

Fig 72. To reduce a pot belly tighten the gluteal muscles (buttocks).

Fig 73. Stand tall and pull your shoulders back just a little for good posture.

caused by muscle weakness, muscle strain, mental stress, poor sleeping habits, among other reasons.

Think tall for better posture. Stand tall, walk tall, sit tall. When you stretch to be as tall as possible, all of the right things happen. The abdominal and lower back muscles tighten. The chest is raised while the abdomen is flattened. However, if your shoulders are round-ed or your head is held forwards, 'standing tall' will not change these. However, when you stand tall, the shoulders are rotated back-wards so that gravity and the large chest mus-cles do not exert as much forwards pull on them. This makes it easier to hold them back.

There is probably no better way to feel like we did when we were younger than to carry ourselves with a good posture.

CHAPTER 15
Taking Care of Yourself While Exercising

A large number of you will no doubt be walking or running for fitness. There are therefore a few things you can do to make your exercise more pleasant and to reduce your chances of an injury.

YOUR SHOES

When you walk into a shop selling sports shoes, the chances are you'll be overwhelmed by the selection and will feel the urge to buy the shoes endorsed by sports celebrities. Superstores may carry hundreds of different trainers from a dozen major manufacturers. And the same goes for most other types of athletic shoes, from walkers and cross-trainers to basketball shoes and football boots.

If there is a shoe shop with special apparatus, such as treadmills with computerized photo equipment for foot analysis, and trained personnel, you may be able to leave the decisions up to the experts. If you don't have such a podiatric luxury you will need to spend a few minutes getting to know your feet and ankles.

Before you go shopping you should get to know your feet and analyse how you will use your new shoes – for walking, running, aerobics, squash, or another sport. Will you be exercising on grass or on concrete? The harder the surface, the greater the shock-absorbing qualities that you will need. Without adequate shock-absorbing qualities you may be setting yourself up for 'shin splints'. So

runners and high-impact aerobics exercisers must think about the quality of the sole.

Just as human feet vary, so do sports and fitness levels. For example, if you only jog a little every week or kick the foot ball around with your grandchild from time to time, an all-purpose cross-training shoe should be fine. But if you do a certain sport or activity three or more times a week, you should wear shoes specific to that sport or activity; they may help you to avoid injuries such as 'shin splints' or ankle sprains.

As we age, our bodies deteriorate. We may still think like 25-year-olds, but our bodies are showing the wear and tear of all those years of living the good life. Even if we have exercised throughout our lives our bodies will become more susceptible to overuse injuries. We therefore must be much more particular to our shoes, the surface on which we exercise, and any warnings our body gives us relative to pain.[1]

In general, people who run or do aerobics need shoes with a lot of impact-absorbing cushioning. Walkers need shoes that have extra shock absorption at the heel as well as soles that provide a good roll off the toes. People who play court sports need shoes that help to keep the ankle stable during side-to-side movements, which means that the sole cannot be too thick.

Which features do you need? To begin with, you should know if your feet have high, medium or low arches. It is easy to tell which kind you have. Just wet the bottom of your bare foot and make a footprint on a hard surface. If the forefoot and heel areas are connected by a mark about an inch wide, you have high-arched feet. If the footprint looks somewhat like the shape of your foot, you have a low arch. A medium arch falls somewhere in between.

For a foot with a high arch, a less flexible foot, you will want a more cushioned sole. If you are flat-footed, your feet are probably too flexible, and you would want a stiffer shoe. Those who have medium arches would want something in the middle – a so-called 'stability shoe'.

Keep in mind any foot problems you have had and try to find a shoe that can accommodate them. Do you have a history of ankle sprains? Then perhaps you should have a high-topped shoe for better ankle support. Have you had deep arch pain? Maybe you need a

special arch support. Do you have bunions? Then you need a shoe with a wide toe box.

Women should be cautious when selecting shoes. Downsized men's shoes have long been offered as 'women's' shoes, and some still are. But their heels can be too loose, which prompts women to wear smaller sizes that can cause problems. Women should seek out shoes that fit their feet properly. Some companies, including Nike, Adidas and Reebok, now offer models specifically designed for women's feet. Saucony is noted for shoes that fit women's feet well, because its shoes tend to have narrower heels. While your new shoes should feel comfortable right away, you should still break them in. Your wider foot may have to stretch the shoe width just a little.

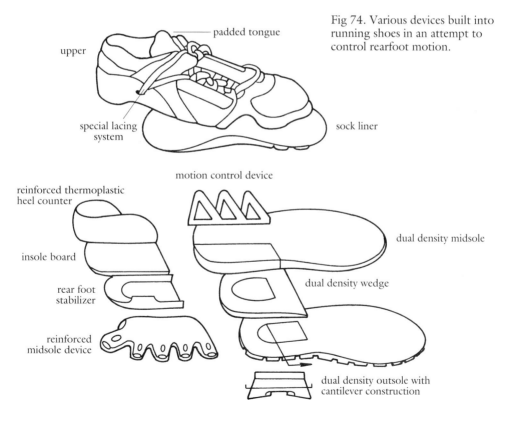

Fig 74. Various devices built into running shoes in an attempt to control rearfoot motion.

padded tongue

upper

special lacing system

sock liner

motion control device

reinforced thermoplastic heel counter

insole board

rear foot stabilizer

reinforced midsole device

dual density midsole

dual density wedge

dual density outsole with cantilever construction

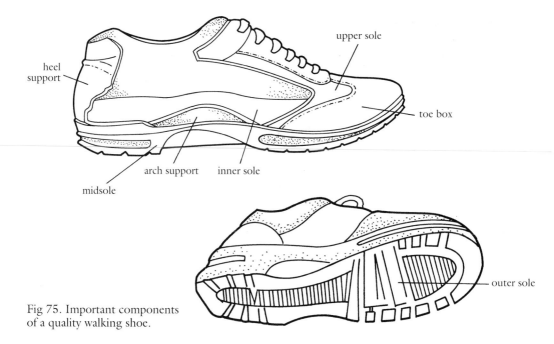

Fig 75. Important components of a quality walking shoe.

Monitor the condition of your shoes as they get older. After about 500 miles (800km) (range from 300miles (480km) to 700 miles (1,130km) depending on the shoe and your own weight), the cushioning on most shoes wears out. However, some of the air-cell shoes and gel cushions may last longer.

Ankle Braces

If your ankles are prone to sprains, it is a good idea to wear ankle braces. This is particularly true when playing court and field games and running on an uneven surface, but even running on a flat surface may create problems – especially if you are running on the pavement and must go up and down kerbs occasionally. Ankle braces can encircle the ankle with a rather stiff cloth which is held tight with laces or Velcro, or they can be open stabilizers with plastic or metal sides. These give the ankle more up and down flexibility, but still stop the sideways movement which causes the sprain. They cost about twice as much as the simpler braces.

An ankle brace which reduces the overpronation of the ankle and foot may assist in preventing overuse injuries.[2]

Checklist for Buying Sport Shoes

- Have your feet measured when they are at their largest: at the end of the day or after a run, walk, game, or practice.
- Wear your workout socks.
- Have both feet measured.
- Try on the shoes, because sizes vary by manufacturer.
- Make sure both shoes fit.
- Ensure that the shoe provides at least one thumb's width of space from the longest toe to the end of the toe box.
- Shoes should also feel comfortable through the arch, fit well across the ball of the foot, and hold the heel firmly.

SPORTS SURFACES

The type of sports surface is also more important as we age. Sand or grass are much more forgiving than asphalt or concrete. They should therefore be much easier on our ageing joints. Another medium is water. You can swim or run in the pool or lake. Running in water, called deep-water running, is done with a weight-supporting life vest. It is found to be even more strenuous than running on the ground, but it doesn't have any negative effects on our bones or joints.[3]

DRESSING FOR THE WEATHER

You will naturally dress according to two factors, the weather and your activity. For example, if you are a cross-country skier you may be out for 4 to 6 hours. You will be working hard, but you don't really want to sweat. Consequently, you will dress in a number of layers. As you warm up, you will remove successive layers so that the cold air will neutralize your body's heat.

On cold days, be certain to dress warmly. More layers are better than one or a few layers because each layer traps air, which is an insulator. It is essential to keep your muscles warm so that they can perform efficiently and not cramp. You will want to avoid the possibility of frostbite or other cold weather problems. Keep your ears, nose, fingers and toes warm. If you are a skier or a mountain climber always keep a mask, hat and gloves handy, and be certain that you have warm socks.

If you are running on a hot day you will want to wear as little as possible so that the perspiration on your skin will evaporate quickly and cool you down.

Excess heat not only negatively affects your performance and comfort, but it can also be a source of serious health problems such as heat exhaustion and sunstroke.

As the outside temperature increases it becomes less and less possible to get rid of the heat of the body which exercise produces. For example, if exercising at 3°C (37°F) you are 20 per cent more effective in eliminating body heat than if you are exercising at 20°C (78°F) and 150 per cent more effective than if you were exercising at 40°C (104°F). It is not uncommon for the body to reach a temperature of 40 to 41°C (104 to 105°F) when exercising. But normal resting body temperature is 37°C (98.6°F). The high heat makes it difficult, or impossible, for the perspiration to evaporate so the body cannot be effectively cooled.

The heat generated in the muscles is released by:

- Conduction – from the warmer muscles to the cooler skin;
- Convection – of the heat loss from the skin to the air; and
- Evaporation – of the perspiration being vapourized.

Conduction

This occurs through the body's liquids, such as the blood, absorbing the heat created by the contraction of the muscles and moving it to the cooler skin. Water can absorb many thousands of times more heat than air can, so blood is an excellent conductor of heat from the muscles.

Convection

This occurs when the heat near the skin is absorbed into the atmosphere. For a swimmer in a cool pool, effective convection is very easy. For the runner it is more difficult. It is aided by a lower air temperature and by wind.

WIND SPEED MPH	WHAT THE THERMOMETER READS (DEGREES F)											
	50	40	30	20	10	0	−10	−20	−30	−40	−50	−60
	WHAT IT EQUALS ON EXPOSED FLESH											
40	26	10	−6	−21	−37	−53	−69	−85	−100	−116	−132	−148
35	27	11	−4	−20	−35	−49	−67	−82	−98	−113	−129	−145
30	28	13	−2	−18	−33	−48	−63	−79	−94	−109	−125	−140
25	30	16	0	−15	−29	−44	−59	−74	−88	−104	−118	−133
20	32	18	4	−10	−25	−39	−53	−67	−82	−96	−110	−121
15	36	22	9	−5	−18	−36	−45	−58	−72	−85	−99	−112
10	40	28	16	4	−9	−21	−33	−46	−58	−70	−83	−95
5	48	37	27	16	6	−5	−15	−26	−36	−47	−57	−68
CALM	50	40	30	20	10	0	−10	−20	−30	−40	−50	−60

Little danger if properly clothed — Danger of freezing exposed flesh — Great danger of freezing exposed flesh

Fig 76. 'Wind-chill' factor.

Wind affects the body temperature by cooling it faster than the registered temperature would warrant. We have all heard of the wind-chill factor present on colder days. The wind makes the body experience more cold than would be expected by the actual temperature. (see chart). But even on warmer days, the wind will evaporate the perspiration and cool the body faster than might otherwise be expected. This may increase the need for fluids to continue the production of sweat. A 4mph (6.4km/h) wind is twice as effective in its cooling properties as is a 1mph (1.6km/h) wind. (This is the basis for the wind-chill factor associated with winds in cool environments.)

Evaporation

This is the most effective method for cooling a body which is exercising in the air. Each litre of sweat which evaporates takes with it 580 kilo-calories. This is enough heat to raise the temperature of 10 litres of water 58°C (2.2gals at 105°F) (ten and a half quarts of water 105°F). As the skin is cooled by the evaporation of the sweat, it is able to take more of the heat from the blood and thereby cool the blood so that it can pick up more heat from the muscles. For this reason, it is not recommended to change to dry clothes when you are sweating on a hot day. As more perspiration is evaporated from your wet clothes you will get a greater cooling effect.

Humidity is the most important factor regulating the evaporation of one's sweat. High humidity reduces the ability of the perspiration to be evaporated. It is the evaporation of the sweat which produces the cooling effect as the perspiration goes from liquid to gas. Exercising in a rubber suit has similar effects to exercising in high humidity because the water cannot evaporate. Rubber suits are therefore not recommended.

REPLACING YOUR FLUIDS

The ingredients of sweat change as you exercise. At the beginning there are a number of salts excreted. Sodium chloride (common table salt) as well as potassium, calcium, chromium, zinc and magnesium salts can be lost. The initial sweat contains most of these salts but, as the exercise continues, the amount of salts in the sweat is reduced because some of the body's hormones come into play. Aldosterone, for example, conserves the sodium for the body. Consequently, the longer we exercise the more our sweat resembles pure water.

A normal diet replaces all of the necessary elements lost in sweat. Drinking a single glass of orange or tomato juice replaces all or most of the calcium, potassium and magnesium that has been lost. Further, most of us have plenty of sodium in our daily diets.

While there are 'fluid replacement' drinks on the market, they are usually not recommended. Water, the most vital element, is slowed in its absorption if it contains other elements such as these salts and sugar. Water alone is therefore the recommended drink for fluid replacement. For those who want to replace water and sugars for energy, the best drinks are those which contain glucose polymers (maltodextrins). So if you are using fluid replacement drinks, check the label. Both caffeine (coffee, tea and cola drinks) and alcohol dehydrate the body so should be avoided.

Adequate fluid is essential to the functioning of an efficient body. When body fluids are reduced by sweating, less fluid is available in the blood and other tissues. These make the body less efficient and, in some cases, can result in serious sickness or even death. To keep the body hydrated, take frequent breaks for fluid intake. However, even frequent breaks seldom give an athlete enough fluid. The thirst does not signal the true need for fluids. It is therefore better to plan sufficient breaks for water and to encourage all athletes to drink more water than they think they need.

Dehydration

Dehydration due to excessive heat and/or inadequate fluid intake can cause serious heat-related illnesses. A sudden change in the heat or humidity, such as occurs when you train or travel to a warmer or more humid climate to compete, can cause problems. If you were to travel to India, Egypt or the Caribbean to compete in a marathon or a football match it would probably take 10 days to 2 weeks to acclimatize yourself to the warmer or more humid climate.

A tennis player may lose 0.5 to 2.5 litres (0.88 to 4.4 pints) of water in an hour. Older athletes, women and those not accustomed to exercising in heat have the biggest problems. As much as 1.5 litres (2.6 pints) of water may be lost before one feels thirsty. It is therefore essential to keep drinking water or other fluid replacement drinks.[4]

Among the changes which will probably occur are: a reduced heart rate (due to less need for blood to heat the skin, resulting in less blood flow to the skin), an increase in the amount of blood plasma, increased sweating, perspiring earlier when exercising, increased salt losses and the psychological adjustments required by the greater heat and humidity.

A comprehensive French study of blood changes during a marathon has indicated that the sodium ions were not significantly reduced and potassium actually increased. This may make us question the need for these in sports drinks. However, the sugars and water in the sports drinks may be necessary. The average marathon runner loses about 4lb (1.8kg) during the race. Most of this is water, with some of it coming from the use of sugars (glycogen) and body fats. (About 2,900 kilocalories are used in a marathon run.) During the run, the body creates some water as it uses the glycogen. About

36oz (1kg) is produced in this process. Urination is also decreased, thereby saving the body's water store.[5]

SKIN PROBLEMS

People who exercise are prone to numerous skin problems caused by increased moisture (athlete's foot), friction (blisters) or damaging elements like cold, sunlight and infection. Most skin problems, however, can be prevented by keeping the skin dry, clean and protected.

Sweating is a common cause of skin problems. Wet skin promotes the proliferation of otherwise normal skin bacteria and other microscopic organisms. Foot odour, for example, is largely due to bacteria that thrive in a moist environment. These same bacteria can also cause pitted keratolysis, a foul-smelling condition in which tiny pits appear on the heels and soles.

'Jock itch' (tinea cruris) and athlete's foot (tinea pedis) also occur more often in moist conditions. Continuing to wear wet clothing after a workout also increases the risk of folliculitis, a bacterial infection of the hair follicles. Infections like impetigo and bacterial folliculitis can also spread via surfaces like padded workout benches and the handles on weight machines. Warm, moist conditions allow these organisms to thrive. Preventing 'jock itch' requires that you keep the skin of the groin as dry as possible. Loose trousers and underwear allow more air to reach these areas. Exercisers should bathe and change clothes (including underwear) as soon as possible after working out. Antibacterial soap can also help to keep the bacteria count down, thorough drying of the skin is also important.

Socks should be absorbent or made of synthetic material that 'wicks' away moisture. Go barefoot or wear sandals when possible to allow your feet to be moisture-free. Your shoes should be allowed to dry for at least 24 hours between uses. Feet should be washed and rinsed well every day, and then thoroughly dried. (A hair drier may help.) In addition, benzoyl peroxide 5 per cent or 10 per cent gel or a spray underarm antiperspirant that contains aluminium chlorohydrate or aluminium chloride can be applied to the feet once or twice daily.

People who have repeated bouts of athlete's foot can apply over-the-counter products such as miconazole nitrate, tolnaftate or clotrimazole to help prevent recurrence.

Friction is another common cause of skin problems. Chafing often occurs in areas where skin rubs on clothing or another skin surface. Blisters typically appear in thicker, pressure-bearing areas such as the palms of the hands and the soles of the feet. Friction from clothing can also cause an irritation, and even bleeding, of the nipples, often called 'jogger's nipples'. Improper shoes or socks can aid in the development of blisters on the back of the heel. Petroleum jelly applied to areas prone to rubbing or chafing can also help – not only for chafing, but for blisters and jogger's nipples as well. Soft, light, smooth fabric should be worn to avoid jogger's nipples. Bras decrease friction, which probably explains why men have jogger's nipples more often than women. Also, plasters can be placed over nipples to reduce friction.

Blisters occur most commonly on the feet because of rubbing between skin and footwear. Shoes should fit well and be gradually broken in before using them in athletic activities. Use the same drying measures described for athlete's foot, because moisture increases friction between skin and fabric. Wearing a thin pair of socks under thicker, more absorbent socks can also decrease friction.

Cold and sun exposure can cause skin problems or aggravate existing conditions. Common weather-related problems include frostbite, dry skin, sunburn and fever blisters.

Those prone to fever blisters should apply a lip balm that contains sunscreen before going outdoors and then reapply it frequently. Very susceptible people may wish to consult their doctor about preventative drugs like acyclovir.

In most situations, sunburn is easily avoided with the use of protective clothing and sunscreen. Hats and clothing made of tightly woven fabric provide fairly good protection against the sun's harmful ultraviolet rays. Caps protect the scalp and, to some degree, the face. Broad-brimmed hats afford additional coverage of the ears. Waterproof sunscreens with a sun protection factor (SPF) of at least 15 should be applied to exposed skin 20 to 30 minutes before going out in the sun.

To prevent frostbite, wear layers of non-restricting clothing in cold weather, paying special attention to the ears, cheeks, nose, fingers and toes. Check yourself regularly for areas of extreme cold or numbness – especially if you have pain that suddenly stops. Also, check your companions' faces and ears frequently for loss of colour or other signs of freezing. Any area of suspected frostbite should be warmed as soon as possible, but do not rub or massage the skin because rubbing may worsen any damage.

Winter dry skin can be minimized by moisturizing the skin. Bathing and showering should be brief and as cool as tolerable, since prolonged exposure to hot water depletes natural skin oils. Use mild 'moisturizing' soaps. After bathing, the skin should be patted, not rubbed, with a towel. Apply moisturizing lotion or cream immediately after bathing and any time the skin feels dry, especially before going outdoors. Direct contact with wool should be avoided because it can irritate dry skin.

OTHER INJURIES

Women are more likely than men to ankle and knee sprains, stress fractures, shin splints and hip problems when running or playing sports which involve running. Men are more likely to injuries to the front of the thigh (quadriceps), plantar fascitis (pain under the foot) or Achilles tendon problems.[6]

Wearing effective braces (such as ankle braces or tennis elbow braces) can reduce your chance of injury. Running on softer surfaces, doing low impact aerobics, or doing 'deep-water running' can also greatly reduce stress and impact-type injuries.

CHAPTER 16
Stress

We all encounter stresses. They may be life-threatening or merely inconveniences. How we handle them can be the difference between being mentally healthy and mentally ill. Life is a forceful teacher. It has a persistent method of presenting the same lesson again and again until we learn it. But we want to learn it as simply as possible!

Stress can be said to be the response which the mind and body make when psychological requirements are too high.[1] For example writing a letter firing an employee and writing a letter to a friend, both experiences in writing, will probably cause different levels of stress. Stress can also be a physical condition, such as the effect of excess cold or heat on the body.

It is not the cause of the stress, as much as the effect of that stress on the individual, which is the major concern. Loud rock music may be pleasant for one person and a terrible noise to another. Giving a speech before an unknown group of people can be either stimulating or unpleasant depending on the situation.

Individuals who think well of themselves may experience less stress. Their positive feelings make them less likely to be overcome by the stressor and they are more likely to feel in control, rather than have the stressor in control. Studies on humans, at the International Centre for Health and Society at University College in London, and studies on baboons, in Kenya's Serengeti, strongly indicate that the higher an individual is in the hierarchy of the society or in one's job classification, the longer the individual lives. It seemed that both a lower-class baboon or a lower-class human had less control over their lives and therefore more life stress. This was true for humans even when other risk factors such as smoking, cholesterol level and blood pressure were controlled. So self-esteem and the ability to control one's life are certainly positive factors and stress reducers.[2]

Many studies have shown the effects of stress, including the lack of control of one's behaviour at work, and the resulting illness. This does not seem to be a recent occurrence. References to a nineteenth-century England's medical schools and the dissection of cadavers showed that the cadavers from lower social class people had much larger adrenal glands than did their higher social class compatriots. This overworking of the adrenal glands can be directly related to the stress they experienced.[3]

> This above all to thine own self be true,
> And it must follow, as night the day,
> Thou canst not then be false to any man.
>
> Shakespeare, *Hamlet*

THE EFFECTS OF UNHEALTHY STRESS ON THE PERSON

Recent literature has emphasized the potential importance that may be attached to psychosocial stress. Chronic stress is expected to increase the risk of premature death both directly through the immune and neuroendocrine systems and indirectly through adverse behavioural responses such as smoking, excessive drinking, and violent behavioural responses to chronic stress may be seen to vary from country to country, as is suggested by variations between countries in national patterns of causes of death. Similarly, any exposure to chronic stress in disadvantaged groups may increase their risk of different causes of death in different parts of Europe.[4]

The mind and body can react to stressors with anxiety, depression, or hostility.[5] These mental reactions can then be transformed into physical diseases such as heart attack, high blood pressure, ulcers, neck and back pains and asthma. Now we find that even cancers and other illnesses are related to a lowering of the immune system – which is a possible result of stress. The role of stress in causing mental diseases has been known longer but its biochemical effects are being more effectively studied today.[6] As we age, the effects of stress seem to multiply. A stress at age 20 experienced at age 50 can result in much greater

---

Holmes-Rahe Scale

This assigns numerical weights to specific life changes. What is your score for the last year?

Rating Life Changes

Life Event	Value	Life Event	Value
Death of spouse	100	Foreclosure of mortgage or loan	30
Divorce	73	Change in responsibilities at work	29
Marital separation	65	Son or daughter leaving home	29
Jail term	63	Trouble with in-laws	29
Death of close family member	63	Outstanding personal achievement	28
Personal injury or illness	53	Wife beginning or stopping work	26
Marriage	50	Beginning or ending school	26
Fired at work	47	Revision of personal habits	24
Marital reconciliation	45	Trouble with boss	23
Retirement	45	Change in work hours or conditions	20
Change in health of family member	44	Change in residence	20
Pregnancy	40	Change in schools	20
Sex difficulties	39	Change in recreation	19
Gain of new family member	39	Change in social activities	18
Change in financial state	38	Mortgage or loan less than £15,000	17
Death of a close friend	37	Change in sleeping habits	16
Change to different line of work	36	Change in number of family get-togethers	15
Change in number of arguments		Change in eating habits	15
with spouse	35	Vacation	13
Mortgage over £15,000	31	Minor violations of the law	11

When too many changes occur in a short period of time it may be wise to seek counselling to assist in adjusting to these changes. Such counselling might avert serious mental or physical problems. A score of 300 points gives an 80 per cent likelihood of a 'stress' disease.

physical changes. Consequently, we need to be increasingly aware of stressful factors in our lives as we age, and either eliminate them or cope effectively with them.

A number of years ago, the Holmes-Rahe scale was developed. It took into consideration a number of life events, both positive and negative and correlated them with diseases. The more events that a person experienced during one year, the more likely it was that diseases would develop. How do you rate? (*See* box p.159.)

Heart attacks during middle age are ten times more common among men than women. We have evidence to suggest that this is caused at least in part by women's hormones. This is probably one factor, but Dr Paul Mills, a psycho-biologist at the University of California at San Diego, has found another significant factor. In measuring two neurotransmitters, epinephrine and norepinephrine, both of which are significant in the sympathetic nervous system, men had twice the amounts that women had. This would mean that high blood pressure and other negative stress-related body reactions could be twice as high in men when experiencing the same stresses as a woman.[7]

Another difference in the effect of stresses between men and women may be in the causes of the stress. Men's levels of stress-induced neurotransmitters increased much more during competitive and intellectual challenges. Women's levels increased more dramatically during stressful personal situations. Studies in Europe (Karolinska Institute in Sweden) and in the United States (Cornell Medical Center) indicate that when husbands and wives have the same types of jobs the men's stress levels tend to drop as soon as they leave the office. Women's levels tend to stay high throughout the evening, probably because of the family responsibilities which continue into the evening.[8]

The Man in the Glass

When you get what you want in your struggle for self,
And the World makes you King for a day,
Just go to the mirror and look at yourself
And see what that man has to say.

For it's not your father or mother or wife,
Whose judgment upon you must pass;
The fellow whose verdict will really count most
Is the man staring back from the glass.

You may be like Jack Horner and chisel a plum,
And think you're a wonderful guy;
But the man in the glass knows you're only a bum,
If you can't look him straight in the eye.

He's the one to please – don't mind the rest –
For he's with you clear up to the end;
And you've passed your most dangerous, difficult test
If the man in the glass is your friend.

You may fool all the world, down the pathway of years,
And get pats on the back as you pass;
But your only reward will be heartaches and tears,
If you've cheated the man in the glass.

Author Unknown

GOOD STRESS AND BAD STRESS

Dr Hans Selye, the Canadian researcher who pioneered research into stress, tells us that there is good stress (eustress, *eu* from the Greek word for 'good') and bad stress (distress). We need stress in our lives, but we want to increase the eustress and decrease the distress. We want to have the excitement of playing a tennis match, reading a stimulating novel, or travelling to a new destination. These are eustresses. We want to eliminate or control the distresses – the long drive to work, the hassles with the people at home, the lack of challenge at our jobs.

Stress is natural for humans. If you don't want any stress, you should have been a rock. Selye once observed that 'Stress is the spice of life'.[9] But as we encounter stress we must be able to cope with it, then, if possible, eliminate the negative stresses.

Our intelligence can aid us in understanding the causes of our distresses and some of the methods which can be used to reduce those stresses. Our intelligence can also help us to find the lifestyles, the careers and the relationships which will yield the greatest amount of eustresses. It is assumed that a 'self-actualized' life, in which a person experiences a great deal of true joy, will make that person immune to the effects of many negative stresses.

Selye also captured the importance of stress in our lives when he wrote: '... man's ultimate aim in life is to express himself as fully as possible, according to his own lights, and to achieve a sense of security. To accomplish this, you must first find your optimal stress level, and then use your adaptation energy at a rate and in a direction adjusted to your innate qualifications and preferences.'[10]

The General Adaptation Syndrome (GAS)

The General Adaptation Syndrome often occurs when we encounter an unwanted stress. There may be three stages to our adaptation to the stress.

Alarm

The first response is alarm. The heart rate increases, the blood pressure rises, breathing becomes more rapid and digestion slows. These reactions are caused when the hypothalamus (located in the centre of the brain) signals the pituitary (the master gland) to release ACTH (adrenocorticotropic hormone). This hormone stimulates the adrenal glands to release other hormones which activate the sympathetic branch of the autonomic nervous system to release the neurotransmitters epinephrine (adrenaline) and epinephrine. The body is then ready for fight or flight – to attack or withdraw.

This alert and ready state can be elicited by any type of surprise – pleasant or unpleasant. A final-second win by your favourite team, an encounter with a mugger, a near accident while driving, or winning the lottery can each start this 'excitement' phase of a eustressful or distressful event.

Resistance Phase

The second stage of the general adaptation syndrome is the calming or 'resistance' stage when your body attempts to get itself back to normal. The body would like to be in a normal state. This we call 'homeostasis.' It may take only seconds or minutes to regain homeostasis for a positive or 'happy' stress or a minor negative stress. Or it may take a long time to get over the stress. A 'Post-traumatic stress syndrome' is such a long-term negative reaction. This might occur when there is a death of a loved one, the loss of a desired job, or a serious or long-term physical injury.

Exhaustion

The third stage of adaptation, exhaustion, may occur if the stress continues for too long. A rat forced to swim to exhaustion repeatedly will eventually give up when put into the water. A person who is daily confronted with heavy stresses, such as a soldier in battle or a policeman in a crime-ridden ghetto, will often succumb to mental exhaustion. This exhaustion can come at the end of a hectic day or after a long period of confronting one or more stresses. Naturally, the longer the period a person is under stress, the greater the potential exhaustion.

OUR HANDLING OF STRESSORS

We may handle stresses by adapting to them, by reducing their effects (coping), or by eliminating them through appropriate thinking and behaviours. If I am a young child and my father continually yells at me I may just accept the fact – adapt to it. If other children in my neighbourhood experience the same kind of parental behaviour I may assume that it is normal and perhaps the negative effects will be small. Here I would be adapting to the stress.

Things to Do Today

1. Get up
2. Survive
3. Go to bed

Both the physical body and the mind can make adaptations to stresses. The body may adjust by a reduced immune function which can result in a lower resistance to diseases and more frequent colds. The person may develop allergies such as asthma, acne and skin rashes. The cardiovascular system may react with higher blood pressure, tightness in the chest or a more rapidly or stronger beating heart. The blood vessels may react by increasing headaches or by slowing the blood flow to the hands and feet, making them feel cold. The muscular system can respond with pains in the back, neck or jaw. The gastrointestinal system can show involvement by diarrhoea, constipation, burping, flatulence or ulcers. The nervous system may show signs such as dizziness, tics, menstrual irregularities, or sleep problems. Psychologically people may react by anger, boredom, depression, hopelessness, irritability, hostility, anxiety, panic, frustration, or fear. The method of adjustment is likely to be inherited, although some people 'learn' their adjustments by imitating others.

Perhaps I spend all of my free time watching television or I use alcohol or other drugs to cope with my unhappiness. These of course would be poor adjustments. Or perhaps I work extra hard to gain my boss's approval or I exercise to reduce my tensions: these would be more effective and healthier methods of coping with the problem.

There are a number of things that you can do to reduce the effects of the stressors or to eliminate them. Many of the positive things that you can do are the same activities which help you to health in every area of your life – physical fitness; an effective sleep and relaxation

---

Coping with Life Threatening Illness[11]

1. Look the illness in the eye. Acknowledge the threat of the danger, then pursue the cure while letting it affect your life as little as possible.
2. Coping is enhanced when people with a similar problem deal with it together. Women in support groups for their cancer problems lived longer than those who were not in such groups.
3. Take it seriously but don't let it take you over. Put it in perspective and take the opportunity to clarify your priorities – projects you wanted to accomplish, friends you want to see, etc.
4. Take control of everything you can and let go of the rest.

---

regimen; sound nutrition; committed social relationships; a positive attitude towards life; meaningful life goals; and a knowledge of how to change behaviour for the better.

Effective Adjustments to Stress

Adjusting effectively to stress can only happen after we have determined whether or not something can be done about that stress. Assume that a person is in a stressful situation. Suppose that the marriage is unhappy. In such a situation, the person should have evaluated the possibilities, looked at the desired goal, then accepted what cannot be changed. Divorce is a possibility. So is marriage counselling. Can this option be effectively raised with the spouse? What if neither person wants to change? The option may then be separation or divorce.

The Chinese character for 'crisis' is composed of two words, one means 'danger,' the other means 'opportunity.' Perhaps this should be our challenge. Or will that create more stress?

Often, we are faced with stress situations to which we *must* adjust by non-action. A policeman gives me a traffic ticket. My boss fires me. My party lost the election. Quite often, we can take affirmative action that will lessen the stress. I might ask for a transfer to another department if there is a personality conflict with a supervisor. I can go to court to fight the traffic ticket. I can work for my political party so that we can win the next election.

Exercise is often overlooked as an effective method of stress reduction. But when one runs, swims or hits a tennis ball, there is some stress reduction. We often see only the physiological benefits of exercise without recognizing its mental effects. But it is known that forceful exercise, especially where hitting or kicking is involved, is an efficient way of reducing the effects of stress. Psychologists often use soft foam-filled bats or boxing

---

When things go wrong, as they sometimes will,
When the road you're trudging seems all up hill,
When the funds are low, and the debts are high,
And you want to smile, but you have to sigh,
When care is pressing you down a bit,
Rest if you must but don't you quit.

Life is queer with its twists and turns,
As everyone of us sometimes learns,
And many a failure turns about,
When he might have won had he stuck it out,
Don't give up though the pace seems slow,
You may succeed with another blow.

Success is failure turned inside out,
The silver tint of the clouds of doubt,
And you never can tell how close you are,
It may be near when it seems so far,
So stick to the fight when you're hardest hit,
It's when things seem worse,
That you must not quit.

Author unknown

---

gloves filled with air as vehicles by which people can take out their frustrations by hitting another person or an inanimate object.

Too often, stress is handled by reaching for a tranquillizer, a sleeping pill or an alcoholic beverage. 'Boy, I need a drink' is often more of a problem than a solution. Pills and booze are not the effective solutions for which most people hope.

We *can* control some areas of our lives and reduce stress in other areas. However, before we can choose the best method of adjusting to a stress we should:

1. Look for the causes of the stress. Is it something that can be changed or is it something

that must be tolerated? Is it a person or a situation? Or is it possible that the problem is me? Do other people react similarly to what I think is the cause of the problem?

2. It is not necessary to 'win' every confrontation. So evaluate your values and goals. Which ones are unimportant? Which are essential? Must I tolerate some stresses in order to accomplish my greater goal?

3. Be positive. Too often, people concentrate on the negative aspects of a situation. The skunk who said, 'I think of my stripe as a racing stripe,' was looking at the positive side of his situation. We often look at our liabilities rather than our assets, our failures rather than our successes. Successful adjust-

---

Negative Methods of Thinking

1. All or nothing. Everything is black or white, no grey. Seldom is anything totally good or totally bad. Some people only see the negatives.
2. Overgeneralization. Taking one situation and applying it to all similar situations: 'I didn't get that job. I'll never get a job.'
3. Discounting what you have done that is good.
4. Blowing things out of proportion, making them larger or smaller than they are in reality.
5. Mistaking emotional feelings for rational thinking.
6. Jumping to conclusions without all of the evidence being in.
7. Assuming that people are thinking or doing things which will affect you, even though you have no evidence.
8. Labelling yourself as a loser, one who can't get things done.
9. Placing too much guilt on yourself or on others. Get a realistic share of the blame based on the evidence.

---

ments require a positive approach to doing something about the stressful situation.

4. Seek advice. A friend or a professional counsellor may be able to give new insights, and certainly will be able to relieve tensions. Talking over a problem is, in itself, a tension reliever.

5. Do one thing at a time. The seconds pass in single file, but they quickly become minutes, hours … and years. When we concentrate on one thing at a time, we will be more likely to approach the stressful situation in a rational manner. We will be more likely to find a satisfying solution.

6. Keep in mind that while each of us has similarities, each of us is unique. Others' problems are not necessarily exactly like our own. But since similarities exist, we may find some possible solutions to our stress problems by reading what others have done in like situations or by attending group therapy such as Alcoholics Anonymous or Gamblers Anonymous, or group therapy led by professionals.

7. Train ourselves to recognize an impending personal crisis. Emotional upsets at work, arguments in our marriages, and break-ups with people with whom we feel close can initiate a mental problem.

8. If we are 'up-tight,' anxiety-producing situations should be avoided. Problems of society on TV, violent films or stress-filled family situations can accent our stresses.

Work can often be a stress reliever, if it allows us to:

- Receive esteem from others.
- Experience real achievement.
- Is meaningful.
- Uses our knowledge and abilities.

(*The Menninger Letter*, July 1995)

Possible Stressors

Following is an outline of a few possible stressors. Each may cause great distress to some people and none to others.

Physical

A lack of oxygen.
Extreme fatigue or tiredness.
An excess of lead or asbestos in the environment.
Too much heat or cold.
A strong wind.
A loud noise, including loud music.
Some chemicals (some acids or alkalis, alcohol).

Biological

An allergic reaction to poison ivy or poison oak.
An upset stomach from the salmonella bacterium.
Any disease, injury or disability.
Hunger or thirst.
Physical problems of ageing.

Mental

A threat or a perceived threat.
Boredom.
Lack of satisfaction of a basic drive (power, love, meaning).
Failure at school or work.
Mental problems of ageing (each age may have its own problems).
Being in a minority group (racial, ethnic, religious, etc.) if you feel discrimination.
Experiencing a loss, such as death or the break-up of a relationship.

Values

Doing something counter to what one's religion holds dear:

Having an abortion when you consider it wrong.

Lying.
Cheating on a test.

Doing something counter to another type of value:

Ordering a second helping when on a diet.
Buying a coat which isn't needed when you are on a tight budget.

Social Relationships

Not having a good friend.
Unhappiness with parents or children (such as alcoholism or drug use).

Economics

Not having enough money.
Having to pay taxes which are too high.

Career

Unhappiness with one's career.
Inability to obtain a job.
Job pressures.
Lack of control and authority on the job.

Political

War or the threat of war.
Injustices carried on by your government or another government.
Being involved in a law suit.

Geographical

Living in a big city.
Living in a ghetto.
Living in a third world country.
Living in an area which is negatively prejudiced against you because of your sex, race, or religion.
Living in a country which is very hot, very cold, or has long dark winters.

What we often need is a holiday, a restful outing or a quiet time, in order to lessen the feeling of anxiety.

THE IMPORTANCE OF RECOGNIZING OUR STRESSES

The diseases listed in chapters 3, 4 and 5 are often brought on by uncontrolled stresses. An unhappy marriage or job situation grates on us and affects our immune systems. Not only are we unhappy, but we are shortening our lives. When we are not happy, we must not accept our fate but must look for the cause or causes of the problem. Then we must look to see whether we can eliminate the problem, adjust to it, or reduce the consequences of the stress placed on our lives.

READING LIST

Benson, Herbert, *Your Maximum Mind*, New York: Times Books, 1987.

Bolles, Richard, *What Color is Your Parachute? A practical manual for job-hunters and career changers*, Berkeley, CA: Ten Speed Press, 1994.

Friedman, Meyer and Rosenman, Ray, *Type A Behaviour and Your Heart.*, Greenwich, CT: Knopf, 1974.

Kabat-Zinn, Jon, *Full Catastrophe Living*, New York: Delacorte Press, 1990.

Needleman, Jacob, *Money and the Meaning of Life*. New York: Doubleday/Currency, 1991.

Selye, Hans, *Stress Without Distress*, New York: Lippincott, 1974.

Selye, Hans, *Stress in Health and Disease.* Reading, MA: Butterworths, 1976.

Self-Test 1

What are the Major Stresses in my Life?

Score 1 to 5 (with 1 meaning 'little or no problem' and 5 being 'the most severe and bothersome')

1. I don't have enough time to do what I need to do. _____
2. Deadlines for jobs at work are problems. _____
3. My friends and family make too many demands on my time. _____
4. I have at least one boss who bothers me a lot. _____
5. My economy is not in good shape – I need more money. _____
6. I don't have time for recreation. _____
7. I don't know what I want to do with my life. _____
8. I am having trouble with my relationship (or finding a relationship). _____
9. I worry about my children. _____
10. (Other problem[s]) _____ bother[s] me a great deal. _____

According to this evaluation the three major stresses in my life are:

1. _____
2. _____
3. _____

Self-Test 2 (Stress symptoms)

Score 1 to 5 (1 being the least amount of problem)

1. I put off doing important things (procrastination). _____
2. I can't slow down my mind. _____
3. I don't sleep well (insomnia). _____
4. My moods change often. _____
5. I always have to be doing something. _____
6. I am tired often. _____
7. I get impatient often. _____
8. I avoid others as often as possible or I am very shy. _____
9. I am often angry. _____
10. I am often very sad. _____

Which three of the above adjustments do you make the most often?

1. _____

2. _____

3. _____

Self-Test 3 (Being under control)

(Developed by Aerobics Research, Dallas, TX. Published by Reebok. Reprinted by permission)

Circle YES or NO to answer the question, then rate the level at which you could manage the stress in the right-hand column from 1 to 100:

1	10	20	30	40	50	60	70	80	90	100
Very uncertain			*Somewhat certain*					*Very certain*		

Might you feel stress?   *If yes, could you manage the stress?*

1. You are trying to concentrate, but you are constantly being interrupted.   YES   NO _____
2. You must perform a very boring task.   YES   NO _____
3. You have been thinking about someone who hurt you in the past.   YES   NO _____
4. You have a neighbour who plays loud music all the time   YES   NO _____
5. You have several things to finish in a very short time.   YES   NO _____
6. You are home by yourself and feel lonely.   YES   NO _____
7. You are in a crowded bus and cannot get to the exit in time for your stop.   YES   NO _____
8. You keep thinking about an unpleasant experience.   YES   NO _____

Self-Test 3 (continued)

9. You have taken on more than you are able to do. YES NO _____
10. You are waiting by the street for someone to pick you up, and you are getting cold. YES NO _____
11. Although you have plenty of time, you are worried that you will be late for an appointment. YES NO _____
12. Your closest has moved away and you feel alone. YES NO _____
13. You are in a room that is extremely hot. YES NO _____
14. You must buy a gift for someone and the stores are closing. YES NO _____
15. You saw someone being robbed and keep imagining that it could happen to you. YES NO _____
16. You must wait for a delivery and you have nothing to do. YES NO _____
17. Your friends keep asking you to do things that you do not have time to do. YES NO _____
18. You must get some prescription drugs, but you can't find a chemist's that is open. YES NO _____
19. You have just spent a good deal of time in a place that is very noisy. YES NO _____
20. Although you have tried your hardest, you have not been able to finish your work. YES NO _____

_____

In which areas are you high or low? How can you improve in your weakest areas?

CHAPTER 17
Coping with Stress

As already mentioned, as we age stresses can affect us more severely because our youthful bodies could deal with them more effectively. Consequently, we must take stress, or the threat of stress, more seriously as we age. While the ideal way to handle unwanted stresses is to eliminate them, this is not always possible. We must therefore learn to handle the stresses with coping skills. These skills can be seen as: relaxation techniques, such as meditation; exercise techniques, such as aerobic dance or swimming; or diversion techniques, such as music or reading.

Coping techniques, which may reduce the effects that distresses have on us, can be:

1. cognitive (from the mind to the body), such as meditation;
2. somatic (from the body to the mind) such as exercise; or
3. behavioural approaches (changing behaviours which are harmful), such as time management.[1]

COGNITIVE TECHNIQUES

Cognitive techniques begin with the mind. It is hoped that by correct thinking, or by 'non-thinking', the body can be relaxed and the tensions of the 'distresses' can be reduced. Among the cognitive techniques are meditation, the relaxation response, hypnosis and thought stopping.

Meditation

Meditation is a type of 'non-thinking' which the Hindus of India have used for thousands of years. It was one of the methods which they used to unite with the Brahman (the oneness of nature). During the 1960s, the Maharishi Mahesh Yogi came to the West and both simplified and popularized the idea of meditation. The Maharishi instructed many people on how to teach his technique. For a fee, a person could be given his or her own private 'mantra'. That mantra was to be repeated while the person breathed deeply. Using this technique for 15 to 20 minutes a day once or twice a day proved to be remarkably relaxing. Researchers at Stanford University, along with other institutions, proved that the techniques of the yogi did, in fact, reduce blood pressure and other symptoms of stress.[2] There is a very different set of physiological responses to meditation or the relaxation response than there is to simple rest.[3]

Dr Herbert Benson, a cardiologist at the Harvard Medical School, acknowledged that transcendental meditation can accomplish many of these relaxation techniques, so he wrote a book called *The Relaxation Response*.[4] He wrote that meditation can be done by almost anyone, without special lessons. It doesn't have to be a religious experience.

His directions are to sit in a comfortable chair in a quiet room. Assume a restful position. Close your eyes. Try to relax all your muscles. Then breathe through your nose and become aware of your breathing. Just think about your breathing, and as you breathe out you say to yourself silently some one-syllable word which can free the mind from logical thought. You might use the word 'one' or 'on' or the Hindu word 'om' which is often used by Yogis as a mantra. The objective of the word is to take away your normal thoughts. Don't use a word like 'sex' or 'money' – they will keep your mind active.

Do this breathing, relaxing and repeating the nonsense word for about 20 minutes. You can open your eyes to check the clock, but it's important that you remain undisturbed for the entire period. Maintain a very passive attitude. Do not worry about how well you are meditating, or you may inhibit the response. If distracting thoughts occur, let them. The meditating word will return naturally.

This relaxation response of Dr Benson's has proved to be extremely effective in lowering blood pressure. Many relaxation therapists say that anxiety or emotional tension and relaxation are mutually exclusive. You cannot be tense if you are relaxed. And it has certainly been proven medically and psychologically that where there is anxiety there is muscle tension. But when muscle tension is relieved, so is the anxiety.

Dr Benson believes that, if we cannot do anything about the stressful lives which so many of us lead, we can at least do something to alleviate the damages of such a life. We can take relaxation breaks. We can do something to relax other than reaching for an artificial aid such as a cigarette, alcohol, or a tranquillizer. We might take naps a couple of times each day, use a meditation technique, or use a type of biofeedback. The effects of relaxation on people with specific medical problems, such as high blood pressure and asthma, have been consistently demonstrated. Once a person can use the relaxation

response it is possible to drop the blood pressure ten to twenty points with only a few breaths. So what Dr Benson had found was that at least one part of meditation was merely the control of the parasympathetic system.

Hypnosis

In hypnosis the mind is taught to relax through the power of suggestion. Some people are quite susceptible to such suggestion. Others are not. Hypnosis should only be done by a trained and licensed therapist.

Thought Stopping

Thought stopping is a technique in which unwanted stress-producing thoughts are removed. The individual imagines a situation in which the negative thoughts might occur. (Dealing with a discourteous customer at work would be an example.) A timer is set for about 3 minutes of this imagining. When the timer indicates that the pre-set time is up, the therapist or the patient yells 'stop'. The individual then keeps his or her mind blank for about 30 seconds. If the thoughts return the patient again says 'stop'.

When the individual has been able to do this with the therapist's help, the process is repeated without the therapist's intervention. The third stage is for the patient to substitute positive and assertive thoughts for the undesired negative thoughts. 'I will relax during the examination', or 'I am prepared for this job', are examples. This method of 'thought stopping' is often effective in eliminating obsessive stress-producing thoughts.

Mental Imagery or Visualization

This technique is common among athletes but it can be used by anyone. It involves imagining yourself doing what you want to do or should do in a certain situation. If you are trying to stop smoking after dinner you may imagine yourself chewing gum or taking a walk after dinner. The imagined action can be influential in having you perform that action after dinner. This technique can be used in thinking of yourself from the outside, such as watching yourself in a movie, or imagining yourself doing the action – from the inside.

For example, if your boss is frequently angry at you with no real reason you may learn to tune him or her out and not react with anger. Just see yourself in that situation. See yourself acting more effectively to reduce the effects of the stressor. If you find that you are shy at social gatherings and would like to be more outgoing, imagine yourself going up to people and starting a conversation. (Most people are just as shy as you are and welcome a chance to talk.) So imagine the different kinds of conversations you can start. Mental imagery is a very simple method of making positive changes to stressors.

SOMATIC TECHNIQUES

Somatic (body to mind) techniques are begun with the body as the focus but the mind relaxes as the body responds to the specific technique. Among the somatic techniques are yoga, progressive relaxation, diaphragmatic breathing, massage, and physical exercise.

Yoga

Yoga is an ancient Hindu method of religious salvation. The Hindus had several yogas (paths) to religious experience. Hatha yoga, the method which is discussed here, is the method in which the body is controlled, usually by stretching and deep breathing. The Hindu would use this as the starting point for mind control (meditation). Most people in the West who use yoga regard it as a relaxing and physical flexibility activity. In using yoga as a relaxation technique, one will gain the ability to stretch tensed muscles and will also get the relaxation advantages of diaphragmatic breathing. There are numerous books and classes which can explain the techniques involved.

Diaphragmatic Breathing

This is simply deep breathing using the diaphragm (the major breathing muscle). Many people do not use the diaphragm properly. They use the auxiliary breathing muscles of the chest and neck. Deep abdominal or diaphragmatic breathing is a method of relaxation which is a part of many other techniques – meditation, relaxation response, progressive relaxation, yoga, swimming, and so on. As such, it has some of the same benefits as these other activities. The usefulness of the technique is that it does not require a great deal of practice and it can be done anywhere and at any time.

To learn the technique, if you do not already know how to do it, merely lie on the floor. Uncover the abdominal area so that you can see the skin between the lower part of the ribs and the hips. As you breathe, see that your abdomen is rising and falling. If your chest, but not your abdomen, is moving up and down you are not using your diaphragm effectively.

Physical Exercise

Physical exercise can help a person to relax in several ways. It can be a recreational pursuit, a rhythmic endurance exercise, or a pleasant, physically fatiguing experience.

A recreational pursuit, such as a game of tennis or golf, a day of downhill skiing or an afternoon of aggressive sailing can make a person forget about the problems which have created the stressful feelings in one's life.

171

A rhythmic activity such as distance swimming, running, walking, rowing or cross-country skiing can provide both the diversion of a recreational activity and the rhythmic breathing of a meditation session. But for such an exercise to have stress reducing effects several factors must be present.

1. It should be enjoyable.
2. It should be aerobic and should not be considered to be competitive by the participant.
3. It should be of moderate intensity and last at least 20 minutes.[5]

While people generally report that they feel better after exercise, not all exercise is equally beneficial. In fact, some exercise can create stress. A competitive runner or swimmer working to exhaustion so that a peak performance can be achieved in the championship meeting is such an example. Similarly, recreational swimmers in uncomfortably warm water show an increase in stress. A golfer or tennis player under pressure to win would be another example.

People who are particularly competitive in life may carry that competitiveness into their recreational pursuits and negate the stress-reducing benefits which would have accrued if the exercise had been truly recreational. It is important that if exercise is to be used to reduce stress it must be pleasant – it must be play. Running may be play for one person but work for another.

Many people have experienced a particularly high level of stress relief after 30 to 50 minutes of aerobic activity. This is often called the 'exercise high' and is suspected to be related to the brain's reaction to increased endorphins – brain chemicals similar to opium.

If an exerciser, particularly an aerobic exerciser, has participated in the exercise several times a week for more than a year, the psychological benefits are greater. It has been found that for runners who had run at least 30 miles a week for two years, a single episode of high intensity work on a treadmill greatly reduced the anxiety level of that person and increased the alpha brain waves (the waves present during meditation). But this same level of exercise for people who were not long-time runners did not produce these same levels of relaxation.[6] These stress-reduction benefits increased as the number of exercise sessions per week and the number of weeks increased. The benefits from the exercise seem to last 2 to 4 hours.[7]

It is obvious that a person who is physically fit will have a better self-concept than one who is unfit. This is an important part of a person's total self-concept and their self-esteem. Since people with better self-concepts and higher self-esteem are more able to handle stressors, physically fit people should experience fewer negative effects from stressors than those who are unfit.[8]

Exercise activities which have positive outcomes for us are more likely to result in better self-concepts. These positive outcomes might be in:

- success (such as running or swimming faster, or losing weight and developing a more pleasing body shape);
- increased feeling of physical competence (such as skiing or playing tennis better), or
- goal attainment (such as lifting a heavier weight, reducing one's resting pulse rate, or shooting a lower golf score).

Effective exercise has also been shown to reduce the illnesses which often accompany stressful events in our lives.[9] Exercisers also report a lower incidence of colon, breast and prostate cancer.[10]

So it can be seen that exercise is both an effective method of *preventing* the stronger negative reactions that can result from stressors and a method for *reducing* those negative reactions when they are present. These are benefits which accrue in addition to the commonly sought outcomes of weight control, aerobic fitness, strength, muscle definition and flexibility.

Exercise has been shown to be as effective as other stress-management techniques in reducing depression, tension and anger.[11] Since exercising aerobically (running, swimming, etc.) is inexpensive and takes the same amount of time as other techniques, while giving additional benefits of weight control and cardiovascular fitness, it should be high on everyone's list of necessary daily activities.

CHOOSING THE COPING TECHNIQUE

Each type of stress may be more effectively handled by the choice of an appropriate coping technique:

- When you are experiencing physical symptoms such as: tense muscles, a rapid heart rate or a lack of energy, a physical activity may help you to better handle the stress. Running, swimming, cycling, cross-country skiing, massage or yoga may be the better choices for your stress reduction.
- When your stress reactions are mental such as: anxiety, worry, insomnia, and negative thinking about yourself, your better choices for coping may be: meditation, the relaxation response, or hypnosis.
- If your stresses are caused by a hectic schedule, having too many things to do and too much responsibility, your better coping mechanisms may be: assertiveness training (to be able to say 'no' to some people who want more of your time), time-management (to be better able to schedule the important activities), biofeedback, and

psychological assistance to change your time-pressured type A behaviour to a more relaxed mode of living.

REDUCING OR ELIMINATING OUR DISTRESSES

The ideal method for handling stresses is not merely to 'cope' with them but rather to eliminate them – if that is a possibility. Often people just accept a stressor rather than find a way to eliminate the problem. *Effective thinking* can often aid us in many areas, and eliminating stressors is one very important area. Also, learning effective thinking will help to raise our level of self-esteem because it is an important aspect of our evaluation of ourselves. We should not get upset because we made a mistake because making a mistake indicates that you at least tried to do something.

Effective decision-making is the sign of a mature, self-actualized person. But how do we think? How do we choose wisely? What are the steps to effective thinking and effective problem-solving? How can we use the proven thinking techniques to reduce or eliminate problems and stresses in our lives?

The Scientific Method of Problem-Solving

The famous American philosopher-psychologist-educator John Dewey can be credited with the approach we will suggest to solving problems. It was his contention that the method of science can be applied to our individual problems; and when applied should make the problems more easy to solve. Here are the steps you might use to solve a problem:

1. Define the problem.
2. Clarify the problem with facts about it.
3. Look at several possible solutions.
4. Choose the best possible solution.

5. Try it and evaluate its outcome.

Successful use of problem-solving can reduce stresses at every age and can even reduce severe depression.[12] But as with most techniques which work, it takes thought, time and commitment. So if you honestly want to make a change in your life, here are the steps.

TAKING CHARGE OF YOUR LIFE

Life never runs completely smoothly. There are always those impediments to happiness – those stressors in our lives. Often people dwell on the stresses. Their whole lives may be used in making excuses or in retreating from life through drugs, deep depressions or other unhealthy escapes.

Our lives will all be touched by some negative stressors – disabilities, failures, death, break-ups of relationships and other personal catastrophes. We cannot let these hurdles trip us and stop our race towards a positive, fulfiling, socially useful life. We must learn how to eliminate those stressors that we can and successfully cope with those which we cannot. As world renowned sport psychologist Tara Scanlan has questioned: 'Do we want to spend our lives coping or enjoying?'

Perhaps the most famous, and the most succinct, phrasing of our task was enunciated by the German theologian Reinhold Niebuhr in what is called 'The Serenity Prayer'

God grant me
The **serenity** to accept the things I cannot change;
The **courage** to change the things I can; and
The **wisdom** to know the difference.

CHAPTER 18

Developing Your Own Positive Health and Fitness Programme

Before you develop your own programme directed at achieving better health, you must be quite certain of why you want to change and how strong your motivation is. If you understand that the saturated fat and cholesterol in egg yolks is bad for most people's hearts and frying the egg makes it far worse, but you love your fried eggs every morning – what will you choose to do? It is YOUR LIFE!

Obviously, every health-directed behaviour you undertake should make you live a little longer and feel a little better. But when healthier behaviour requires that we change our traditional patterns of living it is very difficult. Getting off of the sofa and jogging for 20 minutes, eating whole-grain cereal rather than bacon and eggs for breakfast, or taking time to relax with a meditative type of inactivity are all rather great changes in our life styles. Is it worth it? Would you rather live fast, die young, and have a good-looking corpse?

CHANGING OUR DIET

The major negatives in our diets are too much fat, especially saturated fats, and too many calories. If you are 'salt sensitive' you may also have too much salt in your diet and your blood pressure can be raised because of it.

Getting the proteins you need is simple. The highest quality are in egg whites, skim (non-fat) milk and fish. Fish (especially salmon, trout and herring) have the additional advantage of being able to slow blood-clotting time through their omega 3 fatty acids. It is a good idea to eat fish at least three times a week.

Poultry is the second level of protein in quality. But if you are trying to reduce fat and cholesterol, take the skin off because most of the fats in poultry are in the skin. Organ meats, while they have a good quality of protein and vitamin B_{12}, are very high in saturated fat and cholesterol. And of course steak is the lowest quality of protein of any of the animal products.

Carbohydrates should make up the bulk of your diet. Since most vitamins and minerals are found in the 'complex carbohydrates' it is best to eat the fruits and vegetables (with beta carotene and vitamin C) and the grains and beans (with the B vitamins and E) rather than sweets and chocolate. While either will supply the energy you need the 'simple sugars' do not have the vitamins, minerals and fibres which are present in whole fruits and vegetables.

Fats are almost impossible to avoid. If you are eating fish you will get all the fat you need. The problem with fats is to reduce the total amount. All fats are related to a higher risk of cancers and saturated fats and cholesterols are related to higher risks of heart disease. Also the 'dreaded' free oxygen radicals which are associated with both ageing and many diseases are the result of the breakdown of fats.

When buying foods which have the nutrient content listed on the package, check for the amount of fat. Find the number of kilocalories (total energy) and divide by the number of grams of fat multiplied by nine (calories in a gram). It is best if the percentage of fat calories is under 20 per cent, but definitely keep under 30 per cent.

Also look at the type of ingredients. A fish product may be quite high in fat but if the fat calories come primarily from the fish they are okay. But when you see that the fat comes from animal fat, butter, palm kernel oil or coconut oil – avoid it. Most biscuits and crackers are made with these harmful oils, so check the ingredients or make your own.

Sometimes the ingredients are not on the package but you can be certain that most cakes, pies and pastries are made with butter and eggs. Your arteries can't tell the difference between these 'hidden' fats and those fried eggs which were staring at you from your breakfast plate.

Frying foods is not recommended because fats are generally negatives in our diets. It is best not to fry foods in any type of oil. Butter and lard are the worst vehicles for frying because they are super-saturated with the saturated fats. If you must use an oil, use olive oil or rapeseed oil. But frying in a non-stick pan with no oil is preferable, as you eliminate the harmful fats and reduce calories – sometimes by 50 per cent or more. For example, a potato more than triples its calories when it is fried in a skillet and quadruples its calories in French fries.

Fibres are low in the typical Western diet. You can increase them by eating the skin on your potato, drinking unfiltered orange juice, eating the apple skins and eating whole grains, particularly oats and rice. These fibres can reduce the cholesterol which is absorbed through your intestines and they can reduce the risk of intestinal cancer.

Effective cooking should also be a consideration. Broiling, baking, steaming and boiling are the preferred methods.

Supplementing your diet with vitamin and mineral pills is generally recommended. If you are a vegetarian you will need vitamin B_{12}. We probably all need supplements of the antioxidants: beta carotene, Vitamins C and E, Q 10 and possibly some selenium. Unless your doctor is a specialist in biochemistry and metabolic medicine he or she may not be aware of the current research.

Losing weight may be a concern. Don't try to do it all at once – like the man who chopped off his head to lose 15 ugly pounds quickly. Half a pound or one pound a week is easy to do, especially if you do some aerobic exercise daily. Just remember that a gram of fat contains 9 calories and a gram of alcohol contains 7.

EXERCISE

Flexibility exercises are needed to keep our connective tissues stretched so that our movement is not limited. Since connective tissue shortens very slowly you can get away with doing some toe touching, trunk twisting and ankle stretching once a week. However, if you want to do it daily you should become even more flexible.

Strength exercises should be done to combat the muscle cell loss which we experience with ageing. For thin people, especially women, these exercises are necessary to reduce the chance of developing osteoporosis. Lifting any weight over the head will put some stress on the bones, as well as the muscles. Since bones are an active tissue they need to be forced to do their jobs, that is supporting our bodies. Strength exercises should be done every two days.

If you want to get into a daily routine, you might do some stretching and strength exercises on one day and others on the next. Doing exercises for strength development will have positive effects in reducing any stress which has tightened your muscles. If you tend to get a stiff neck or tight upper back muscles you can do exercises for those areas daily.

Aerobic exercise, or exercise for heart, lungs and blood (cardiorespiratory), is the most important type of exercise for lowering your body weight and your blood fats (triglycerides) and increasing the amount of the 'good cholesterol' or HDL. It is also a great way to reduce mental stresses. Swimming is an outstanding full body exercise. So is cross-country skiing. The skiing, of course, gets you out in nature which can have some additional stress-reducing benefits. Running through the woods or a park can also add that extra perk of communing with nature.

Make your exercise enjoyable. If you like to walk – walk. If you like to play golf – play golf. If you like to watch television – do it while riding your exercise bike. The point is that you can take half an hour out of your day or you can exercise while you are doing what you would have done anyway – such as reading or watching the television.

While running, swimming, cycling or skiing are methods of obtaining maximum fitness, the work of Dr Steve Blair shows that you don't have to do an excessive amount of exercise just to increase your lifespan. Just work in half an hour of some sort of exercise daily. Walk, garden, clean the house, or just about anything else that gets you out of your chair will help.

REDUCING STRESS

As seen in the chapter on ageing, uncontrolled stress is a negative factor in our ageing process because it reduces our immune system while also lowering our contentment level in life. The first thing to do is to eliminate the stress. If the problem is at work: talk to the person who is causing the problem, change jobs in the company, or move to a different company. Sometimes it is not the job situation but rather the job itself. If structural engineering is no longer fun, perhaps you can change to another type of engineering or teach engineering. If that doesn't sound good, you may be able to train for another job which seems more enjoyable.

When you cannot eliminate the stressful situation you should be able to reduce the effects on your body and mind. Meditation, physical exercise, or finding a new type of recreation (painting, cooking, making clothes or reading poetry or literature) may be an answer. Therapy may also help, as will seeing old friends.

YOUR MENTAL AND PHYSICAL FITNESS LEVEL

One thing is certain about us ageing humans – we have the intelligence and the capacity to make positive changes in our lives. The scientific knowledge is there. We merely need to take what we want from that knowledge, then apply it to our lives. The results will be a happier, more fulfiling and longer life. We can sit in our rocking chairs and appear to be busy rocking – but we wouldn't be going anywhere. If we are going to go somewhere, we have to get up and DO!

INTERNET SITES

The following were compiled by Dr Stephen Seiler. Check his sites on the Internet for articles on endurance and updates on sites of interest. He is an exercise scientist with a special interest in endurance sports. Some of these may give you information you need to find out more about your health or to find a 'master's' level group with whom you can exercise: **http://krs.hia.no/ stephens/ index.html**.

Endurance Athletes

- **http://www.medfacts.com/** MED FACTS OF SPORTS Includes both direct readable info and access to an interactive resource on injury diagnosis.
- **http://www.scp.com** MedScape For medical professionals and interested others.
- **http://healthnet.ivi.com/** The OnLine Health Network from the Mayo Clinic.
- **http://www.aeivos.com/** Aeivos Home Page. If you are interested in the issue of ageing in general, and not just your own, this is a great site. They offer a tremendous resource of references related to research in ageing. Plus, there are links to a whole lot more. An academic resource.
- **http://sln.fi.edu/biosci/heart.html** The Heart: An Online Exploration.
- **http://www.amhrt.org/** The American Heart Association Home Page. Both specific and general information.
- **http://www.cdc.gov/cdc.html** The Center for Disease Control. American Tax Dollars at work. There is a lot of information to be found here.
- **http://www.fda.gov/fdahomepage. html** The Food and Drug Administration (FDA). More tax dollars at work.

Exercise Physiology and Sports Medicine

- **http://www.gssiweb.com/index.html** The Gatorade Sports Science Institute. Gatorade does not need to pay for research any more to sell its products, but it still does, and it has a great website to help spread the facts on exercise and performance. Top scientists write for this site.
- **http://www.sportsci.org** Sport Science. One of the best places on the net if your interest is human performance research. It is loaded with resources.
- **http://www.physsportsmed.com/** The Physician and Sportsmedicine (not the magazine). This site can be a good resource on injuries and more.
- **http://www.nismat.org/index.html** The Nicholas Institute of Sports Medicine and Athletic Trauma. This is a nice site with some good reviews on muscle contraction and cardiac function along with a lot of other material. From the famous Lennox Hill Hospital in New York.
- **http://www.clark.net/pub/pribut/ spsport.html** Dr Pribut's Sports Injury Page.
- **http://riceinfo.rice.edu:80/~jenkins/** Dr Jenkins SportsMedWeb. More good sports medicine tips for the endurance athlete.
- **http://rohan.sdsu.edu/dept/coachsci/ intro.html** Coaching Science Abstracts. A monthly listing consisting primarily of article summaries related to training, overtraining, specificity and so on, complete with their interpretation of the data. This is an excellent resource, but if you are serious, read some of these research articles for yourself.
- **http://www-neuromus.ucsd.edu/Mus-Intro/Jump.html** Physiology of Muscle. An excellent source of basic physiology information. They go deeper than this book, for those who want more basic physiology and muscle function information.
- **http://www.tahperd.sfasu.edu/links 3.html** Kinesiology/Health Science Links. A good academic resource.
- **http://www.inect.co.uk/nsmi/** The National Sports Medicine Institute in Great Britain.

- http://indy.radiology.uiowa.edu/Providers/Textbooks/rad/books/MuscleInjuries/MuscleInjuries.html Muscle Injuries, from the Virtual Hospital.
- http://www1.pitt.edu/~pahnet/ The Physical Activity and Health Network. This is a good and growing academic resource from the University of Pittsburgh. Also includes a Japanese version.
- http://www.genome.ad.jp/kegg/metabolism.html Metabolic Pathways. Heavy science.

Sports Nutrition

Much of the nutrition information (read 'advertising') is not of scientific value – merely 'come ons' for the unsuspecting!

- http://www.sfu.ca/~jfremont Jean Fremont's Food, Nutrition and Culinary Arts page. Good nutritional information from dietician and professor Jean Fremont at Simon Frasier Univ. in Canada.
- http://www.nal.usda.gov/fnic/foodcomp/ Nutrient Data from The US Department of Agriculture. This is an outstanding resource for full nutrient information on most foods that you eat.

Cycling

- http://www.halcyon.com/gasman/ Cycling Performance Tips. A nice site from Richard Rofurth M.D.
- http://sunwww.informatik.uni-tubingen.de:8080/sport/rad/rad.html A German cycling site with some nice European history and race results. Lots of Links. It is written in English.
- http://www.cs.purdue.edu/homes/dole/bike.html The WWW Bike Lane. An excellent list of sites, including some great photos.

- http://www.uwm.edu/People/tjbrooks/bauer/bauer.html Team Bauer. Endurance Training for Cyclists.
- http://wwwmath.science.unitn.it/Bike/ Trento Bike Pages. Based in Italy. A great and growing collection of stories and info on road and MTB trips throughout Europe.
- http://www.microship.com/ Nomadic Research Labs. This site describes the science and adventurous spirit behind an eleven year odyssey on the Behomoth bicycle plus much more. Computer Technology merges with Human Muscle Power.
- http://www.go-interface.com/majtaylor/index.html Major Taylor's News and Results Service. For folks who hunger for information on the international racing scene. If you know who Major Taylor was, then you need this site.
- http://home.earthlink.net/~durer/fgf/ Fixed Gear Fever. This is *the* site for track cyclists. But even if you have never been in a velodrome, check out the great photos!
- http://www.cycling.uk.com

Rowing

- http://info.ox.ac.uk/~quarrell/index.html Rachell Quarrell's Rowing Web. If you are a rower you probably know about this comprehensive listing of Rowing Websites; also lists shopping opportunities.
- http://www.rowersresource.com/ The Rowers Resource. A new US-based page. Has results of Olympic selection trials, collegiate races and information about National Team members. This will probably be one of your best bets for rapid rowing results during the Olympics.
- http://www.yampa.com/sports/rowing/ US Women's Sweep Team. This site is maintained by one of the team members. It includes an example of their training regimen.

- http://www.tiac.net/users/rowasone/index.html ROW as ONE. This is a master's rowing camp programme that started just for women but now includes men. You should check out this page if you are in the US.
- http://www.swidoc.nl:8080/english/english.html#bit/" Heinks Rowing Information. This is a nice page based out of the Netherlands. Focus is on Elite Rowing.
- http://www.concept2.com/ Concept 2's home page. Some good basic information on ergometer workouts for new rowers.
- http://users.ox.ac.uk/~quarrell/REGATTA/index.html Regatta Online. The electronic version of the British magazine, *Regatta*.

Running

- http://www.runningnetwork.com/rn/rngjournal/tips/index.html Running tips from the *Running Journal*. An interesting collection of articles.
- http://members.aol.com/trackceo/index.html The Master's Track & Field Page.
- http://members.aol.com/masterstf/records.html Master's Track & Field Records. A current listing of top marks from all over the world for veteran (over 40) runners.
- http://asgard.cbi.msstate.edu/faculty/pearson/masters.html Age-adjusted Running Tables. Where do you stand relative to your same-age peers? 1,500m up to marathon. Percentile rankings, based on top performance in each age group.
- http://www.halhigdon.com/run.html Hal Higdon On the Run. On-line articles from the popular *Runner's World* writer.
- http://website.flash.net/~race26/50dc/index.html 50 States Marathoners. The minimum requirement for inclusion in this elite group is a completed marathon in each of the fifty US States, but some have gone far beyond this!
- http://www.sirius.on.ca/running/vo2.shtml#anchorcal/ Calculate your VO_2 Max. This page has an automatic form for estimating your VO_2 max from running time in any of several distances. It is based on research by a physiologist who has focused on runners for years. Probably a pretty good estimate if you are an experienced runner.
- http://www.win.tue.nl/win/math/dw/personalpages/remkor/athletics/index.html Track and Field Index. Remo, in the Netherlands, is the Web Magnet for all things numerical in running. Record listings by country, lane of the track and so on! Plus much more.
- http://fox.nstn.ca/~dblaikie Ultramarathon World–Dave Blaikie. For you people who run further than 26.2 miles!
- http://storm.cadcam.iupui.edu/drs/drs.html The Dead Runners Society. Runners talking about running. This is a list worth signing on to.
- http://www.ausport.gov.au/aths Athletics Australia. The official site for Australian track and field.
- http://www.runnersworld.com/ Runner's World Online. The most redeeming feature for the Web version is that the news is more timely, and they do report Master's happenings.
- http://www.holmes.gpm.demon.co.uk. Complete runners' network.

Swimming

- http://rohan.sdsu.edu/dept/coach-sci/swimming Swimming Science Journal. An on-line offering from the authors of *Coaching Science Abstracts*. This site will focus on swimming and coaching science.

- http://www.jmeldrum.demon.co.uk Competitive masters' swimming.
- http://www.hk.super.net/~kff/wmswr .html Master's Swimming World Records This link is within World Master's Swimming.
- http://ourworld.compuserve.com/ homepages/swim/homepage.htm Dunwoody Aquatic Master's Page (DAMP). Check out the 2% Club.

Cross-Country Skiing

- http://www.weblab.com/xcski/ skinews.html Cross-Country Skiing News.
- http://www.ussa.org/ The United States Skiing Association.
- http://www.danenet.wicip.org/mad-nord/links.html Nordic Skiing Links.
- http://www.weblab.com/xcski/journal.html Cross-Country Ski World Educational Journal. A good place to go for beginners, as well as advanced skiers.
- http://www.allshop.com/cedro/ archive/chat/CrossCountrySkiing/group.html Sports Chat Sports Site.

Strength Training

- http://www.west.net/~staley/welcome.html Fundamentals of Strength Training for Sport. A resource page for athletes and coaches by Charles Staley.
- http://www.tgx.com/cpu/related. htm Powerlifting Related Sites.

Tennis

- ttbanner.gif at http://www.tennis. org.uk Complete Tennis coverage.

Other Sites of Interest

- http://www.iaaf.org/ The International Amateur Athletics Federation. The site for the international governing body for track and field (athletics). Results, research, subscriptions and so on.
- http://www.triathlon.org/ International Triathlon Union. Governing body for the triathlon. Good results and ranking listings.
- http://www.triathletemag.com/new/ Triathlete Magazine. Current Age Group rankings for the top US duathletes and triathletes.
- http://www.olympic.org/ International Olympic Committee Home Page.
- http://outside.starwave.com:80/outside/online/index.html Outside Online. Any commercial site that covers the US Olympic Rowing Trials and Boston marathon (LIVE) in one day is a great site.
- http://www.stevenscreek.com/ Stevens Creek Software. Sells a computerized training diary that is great (free demo version), books for athletes, and so on.
- http://www.fca.org The Fellowship of Christian Athletes Home Page.

References

Chapter 1

1 Shephard, R.J. *et al.*, 'Personal health benefits of Masters athletics competition', *British Journal of Sports Medicine*, 29, pp. 35–40.

2 Muldoon, M.F. 'What are quality of life measurements measuring?', *British Medical Journal* (hereafter *BMJ*), Feb. 1998, 316, pp. 542–45.

3 Positio statement of World Health Organization presented at the World Congress of Sports Medicine, Orlando, FL., 3 June, 1998.

Chapter 2

1 Pahor, M. & Applegate, W., 'Geriatric medicine', *BMJ*, 315 (7115), 25 Oct. 1997, pp.1,051–71.

Chapter 3

1 Smith, G. D. *et al.*, 'Lifetime socioeconomic position and mortality: prospective observational study', *BMJ*, 314, Feb. 1997, p.547.

2 Kunst, A. *et al.* 'Occupational class and cause specific mortality in middle-aged men in 11 European countries: comparison of population based studies', *BMJ*, 316, p.7, 1636–42 (1998).

3 Meyer, K. *et al.*, 'Effects of exercise training and activity restriction on 6-minute walking test performance in patients with chronic heart failure', *American Heart Journal*, 33 (4), Apr. 1997, pp.447–53.

4 *American Journal of Hypertension*, vol. 5 (8), August 1992; *Journal of American Medical Association.*, vol 268 (21), 2 Dec. 1992.

5 Spina, R.J. *et al.*, 'Exercise training enhances cardiac function in response to an after load stress in older men', *American Journal of Physiology*, 272 (2 pt 2), Feb. 1997, 995–1,000.

6 Ponjee, G.A. *et al.*, 'Regular physical activity and changes in risk factors for coronary heart disease: a nine months prospective study', *European Journal of Clinical Chemistry and Clinical Biochemistry*, 34 (6), June 1996, pp.477–83.

7 Morris J.N., *et al.*, 'Exercise in leisure time: coronary attack and death rates', *British Heart Journal*, 63 (6), June 1990, p.325.

8 *University of California Wellness Letter*, May 1994, p.5.

9 Sparrow D., Dawber T.R., 'The influence of cigarette smoking on prognosis after a first myocardial infarction: a report from the Framingham study', *J Chronic Disease*, 31 (6–7), 1978, 425–32.

10 *Type A Behavior and Your Heart*, New York: Alfred A. Knoph, 1974.

11 *Harvard Health Letter*, 2 (5), Jan. 1992, p.1.

12 Markovitz, Jerome, *et al.*, 'Physiological predictors of hypertension in the Framingham study', *Journal of American Medical Association*, 270 (20), 24 Nov. 1993, p.2,439.

13 *University of California Wellness Letter*, May 1994, p.5.
14 Rayman, M.P., 'Selenium: a time to act', *BMJ*, 314 (387), Feb. 1997, Editorial.
15 'Is alcohol good for the heart?', *Johns Hopkins Medical Letter – Health After 50*, 4 (8), Oct. 1992, p.3.
16 Margolis *et al.*, *Coronary Heart Disease*, Johns Hopkins White Papers, Baltimore, MD: Johns Hopkins Medical Institutions, 1993, p.20.
17 *Ibid.*, p.5.
18 *Ibid.*, p.5.
19 Reported in *Harvard Women's Health Watch*, Oct. 1994, p.6.
20 Hodis, Howard,. 'Circulation', *American Heart Association*, July 1994.
21 'Depression, anger, and the heart', *Harvard Heart Letter*, Feb. 1993, p.7.
22 Hertog, Michael, *et al.*, 'Dietary antioxidant flavinoids and the risk of coronary heart disease', *Lancet*, 342 (8,878), 23 Oct. 1993, p. 1,007.

Chapter 4

1 'Breast cancer genes', Women's Health Watch [Harvard University], 2 (4), Dec. 1994, p.1.
2 Slattery, Martha and Kerber, Richard. 'A comprehensive evaluation of family history and breast cancer risk', *Journal of the American Medical Association*, 270 (13), 6 Oct 1993, p.1563.
3 Colditz, Graham, 'Family history from the nurses' health study', *Journal of the American Medical Association*, 270 (3), 21 July 1993, p.338.
4 *University of California Wellness Letter*, 10 (6), March 1994, p.1.
5 Women's Health Advocate, April 1995, p.7.
6 *Tufts University Diet and Nutrition Letter*, 12 (9), Nov. 1994, p.7.

Chapter 5

1 *Johns Hopkins Medical Letter*, Nov. 1992, p.7.
2 *Johns Hopkins Medical Letter*, Nov. 1992, p.3.
3 *University of California Wellness Letter*, 11 (3) Dec. 1994, p.1, reporting on a study by Maureen Jensen in the *New England Journal of Medicine*, July 1994.
4 *Journal of American Medical Association*, 268 (1), 1 July 1992.
5 Papers presented at the 53rd Annual Meeting of the American Diabetes Association, June 1993.
6 *Johns Hopkins Medical Letter*, Sept. 1994, p.4.
7 *University of California Wellness Letter*, July 1993, pp.4–5.

Chapter 6

1 Lemon, P.W., and Proctor, D.N. (1991). 'Protein intake and athletic performance', *Sports Medicine*, 12, 313–25.
2 Tarnopolsky, M.A., Atkinson, S.A., MacDougall, J.D., Chesley, A., Phillips, S. and Schwarcz, H.P. (1992), 'Evaluation of protein requirements for trained strength athletes', *Journal of Applied Physiology*, 73, pp.1,986–95.
3 Lemon, P.W., Tarnopolsky, M.A., MacDougall, J.D. and Atkinson, S.A. (1992), 'Protein requirements and muscle mass/strength changes during intensive training in novice bodybuilders', *Journal of Applied Physiology*, 73, pp.767–75.
4 FAO/WHO: *Energy and Protein Requirements*, FAO Nutrition Report No. 52; Who Tech. Report No. 522, Rome and Geneva, 1973; FAO/WHO: *Amino Acid Content of Foods and Biological Data on Proteins*, No. 24. Rome, 1970.
5 Sola, R., Motta, C., Maille, M., Bargallo, M.T., Boisnier, C., Richard, J.L. and Jacotot, B, 'Dietary monounsaturated

fatty acids enhance cholesterol efflux from human fibroblasts. Relation to fluidity, phospholipid fatty acid composition, overall composition, and size', of HDL3. *Arteriosclerosis and Thrombosis*, 13, 1993, pp.958–66.

6   Shahar, E., 'A putative role of dietary omega-3 polyunsaturated fatty acids in oxidative modification of low density lipoprotein', *Prostaglandins, Leukotites, and Essential Fatty Acids*, 48, 1993, pp.397–9.

7   Kubow, S., 'Lipid oxidation products in food and atherogenesis', *Nutritional Review*, 51, 1993, pp.33–40. *American Journal of Clinical Nutrition*, 56, pp.499–503.

8   Clark, R. *et al.*, 'Dietary lipids and blood', BMJ, Jan. 1997, 314, p.112.

9   Willett, W.C., Stampfer, M.J., Manson, J.E., Colditz, G.A., Speizer, F.E., Rosner, B.A., Sampson, L.A. and Hennekens, C.H., 'Intake of trans-fatty acids and risk of coronary heart disease among women', *Lancet*, 341, 1993, pp.581–5.

10 Lichtenstein, A.H., Ausman, L.M., Carrasco, W., Jenner, J.L., Ordovas, J.M. and Schaefer, E.J., 'Hydrogenation impairs the hypolipidemic effect of corn oil in humans', *Arteriosclerosis and Thrombosis*, 13, 1993, pp.154–61.

11 Blankenhorn, D.H. and Hodis, H.N., 'Atherosclerosis – reversal with therapy', *Western Journal of Medicine*, 159, 1993, pp.172–9

Reference

Pennington, Jean, Church, Helen. *Food Values of Portions Commonly Used*. New York: Harper & Row, 1994.
(This is essential for anyone seriously interested in nutrition. It lists nearly every food and notes protein, fat and carbohydrate contents, ten vitamins and nine minerals, as well as many other specialized lists of nutrients.)

Chapter 7

1   Hornig, D., and Strolz, F., 'Recommended dietary allowance: support from recent research'. *Journal of Nutritional Science and Vitaminology*, Tokyo, Spec No., 1992, pp.173–6.

2   Witt, E.H., Reznick, A.Z., Viguie, C.A., Starke-Reed, P. and Packer, L., 'Exercise, oxidative damage and effects of antioxidant manipulation', *Journal of Nutrition*, 122, (3 Supplement), 1992, pp.766–73.

3   Kanter, M.M., Nolte, L.A. and Holloszy, J.O., 'Effects of an antioxidant vitamin mixture on lipid peroxidation at rest and postexercise', *Journal of Applied Physiology*, 74, 1993, pp.965–9.

4   Menzel, D.B., 'Antioxidant vitamins and prevention of lung disease', *Annals of the New York Academy of Science*, 669, 1992, pp.141–55.

5   Blass, J.P., Sheu, K.F., Cooper, A.J., Jung, E.H. and Gibson, G.E., 'Thiamin and Alzheimer's disease', *Journal of Nutritional Science and Vitaminology*, Tokyo, Spec No., 1992, pp.401–4.

6   Tallaksen, C.M., Bohmer, T., and Bell, H, 'Blood and serum thiamin and thiamin phosphate esters concentrations in patients with alcohol dependence syndrome before and after thiamin treatment', *Alcohol and Clinical Experience and Research*, 16, 1992, pp.320–5. Darnton-Hill, I. and Truswell, A.S., 'Thiamin status of a sample of homeless clinic attenders in Sydney', *Medicine Journal of Australia*, 152, 1990, pp.5–9.

7   Smidt, L.J., Cremin, F.M., Grivetti, L.E. and Clifford, A..J., 'Influence of thiamin supplementation on the health and general well-being of an elderly Irish population with marginal thiamin deficiency',

Journal of Gerontology, 46, 1991, pp.M16–22.

8 Suboticanec, K., Stavljenic, A., Schalch, W. and Buzina, R., 'Effects of pyridoxine and riboflavin supplementation on physical fitness in young adolescents', *International Journal of Vitamin Nutritional Research*, 60, 1990, pp.81–8.

9 Soares, M.J., Satyanarayana, K., Bamji, M.S., Jacob, C.M., Ramana, Y.V. and Rao, S.S., 'The effect of exercise on the riboflavin status of adult men', *British Journal of Nutrition*, 69, pp.541–51. Winters, L.R., Yoon, J.S., Kalkwarf, H.J., Davies, J.C., Berkowitz, M.G., Haas, J. and Roe, D.A. , 'Riboflavin requirements and exercise adaptation in older women', *American Journal of Clinical Nutrition*, 56, 1992, pp.526–32.

10 Christensen, H.N., 'Riboflavin can protect tissue from oxidative injury', *Nutritional Review*, 51, 1993, pp.149–50.

11 McCully, K.S. 'Homocysteine, folate, vitamin B6 and cardiovascular disease'. *Journal of the American Medical Association* (JAMA), 279, 1998, pp.392–3; Rimm, E.B. *et al.* 'Folate and vitamin B6 from diet and supplements in relation to risk of coronary heart disease in women', JAMA, 279, 1998. pp.359–64.

12 Kimura, M., Itokawa, Y. and Fujiwara, M., 'Cooking losses of thiamin in food and its nutritional significance', *Journal of Nutritional Science and Vitaminology*, Tokyo, 36, (Supplement 1), 1991, pp.S17–24.

13 Salonen, R. *et al.*, 'Vitamin C deficiency and risk of myocardial infarction: prospective population study of men from eastern Finland', BMJ. March 1997, 314 p.634.)

14 Schectman, G., 'Estimating ascorbic acid requirements for cigarette smokers', *Annals of New York Academy of Science*, 1993, pp.686, 335–46.

15 Tuovinen, V., Vaananen, M., Kullaa, A., Karinpaa, A., Markkanen, H. and Kumpusalo, E., 'Oral mucosal changes related to plasma ascorbic acid levels', *Proclamations of the Finnish Dental Society*, 88 (3–4), 1992, pp.117–22.

16 Haymes, E.M., 'Vitamin and mineral supplementation to athletes', *International Journal of Sport Nutrition*, 1 (2), 1991, pp.146–69.

17 Ng, H.T., Chang, S.P., Yang, T.S., Cho, M.P. and Wei, T.C., 'Estradiol administered in a percutaneous gell for the prevention of postmenopausal bone loss', *Asia Oceania Journal of Obstetrics and Gynaecology*, 19, 1993, pp.115–9.

18 Campos, P.M.M., Munoz, T.M., Escobar, J.F., Ruiz de Almodovar, M. and Jodar, G.E., 'Bone mass in females with different thyroid disorders: influence of menopausal status', *Bone Minerals*, 21, 1993, pp.1–8.

19 Matkovic, V., and Ilich, J.Z., 'Calcium requirements for growth: are current recommendations adequate?', *Nutritional Review*, 51, 1993, pp.171–80.

20 Bingham, S.A. et al 'Phyto-oestrogens where are we now?' *Brit. J of Nutrition* May, 1998, 79(5) 393–406; Willard, S.T. and Frawley, L.S. 'Phytoestrogens have agonistic and combinational effects on estrogen-responsive gene expression in MCF-7 human breast cancer cells', *Endocrinology*, Apr. 1998, 8(2), 117–121); Clarkson, T.B. 'The potential of soybean phytoestrogens for postmenopausal hormone replacement therapy,' *Proc. Soc. Exp. Boil. Med.* Mar. 1998, 217(3) 365–8).

185

Chapter 8

1 Maughan, R.J., 'Factors influencing the restoration of fluid and electrolyte balance after exercise in the heat', *British Journal of Sports Medicine*, 31, 1997, pp.175–82.

Chapter 9

1 Cooper, Ken, The Antioxidant Revolution, Nashville, TN: Thomas Nelson Inc., 1994, p.119.

2 Pahor, M. and Applegate W.B., 'Recent advances: geriatric medicine', *BMJ*, 315 (7115), p.1071.

3 Z'Brun A. 'Ginkgo – myth and reality', *Schweiz Rundsch Med Prax*, 84 (1), 3 Jan 1995, pp.1–6.

4 Cited in *BMJ*, 25 Oct 1997 from: *Journal of the American Medical Association*, 278, 1997, pp.1,327–32.

5 Cooper, *op. cit.* in note 1.

6 *Ibid*.

7 Pahor, *op. cit.* in note 2.

8 Cooper, *op. cit.* in note 1.

9 Kristenson *et al.*, *BMJ*, March 1997, 314, p.7,081.

10 Karlsson, J., *Antioxidants and Exercise*, Champaign, IL: Human Kinetics, 1997, p.63; Halliwell, B. and Gutterudge, M., 'Oxygen free radicals and iron in relation to biology and medicine: Some problems and concepts'. *Arch. Biochem.*, Biophys. 246, 1986, pp.501–14; Alessio, H.M. *et al.*, 'Evidence that DNA damage and repair cycle activity increases following a marathon race', *Medical Science in Sport and Exercise*, 22, 1990, p.751; Alesio, H.M., 'Exercise-induced oxidative stress', *Med. Sci. Sports Exerc.*, 25, 1993, pp.218–24.

11 Karlsson, J., 'Advances in Nutrition for High-Intensity Training', Presentation at the World Congress of Sports Medicine, Orlando, FL, 3 June 1998.

12 Karlsson, *op. cit.* in note 10, p.105.

13 Rayman, M.P., 'Selenium: a time to act', *BMJ*, 314 (387) Feb. 1997, Editorial.

14 Karlsson, J., *op. cit.* in note 10, pp. 169, 170.

15 Skjervold, H., 'Lifestyle diseases – human diet', *Meieriosten*, 19, pp.527–9.

16 Drinkwater, B., 'Osteoporosis', Presentation at the World Congress of Sports Medicine, Orlando, FL, 2 June 1998.

17 Reilly, T., Maughan, R., Budgett, R., 'Melatonin: a position statement of the British Olympic Association', *British Journal of Sports Medicine*, 322, June 1998, p.99.

Chapter 10

1 *Los Angeles Times*, 15 July 1994.

2 Shaper, A.G., 'Body weight: implications for the prevention of coronary heart disease, stroke, and diabetes mellitus in a cohort study of middle aged men', *BMJ*, May 1997, 314, p.1,311.

3 McGinnis, J. Michael, 'Actual causes of death in the United States', *Journal of American Medical Association.*, 270 (18,513), 10 November 1993, pp. 2,207–12.

4 American Cancer Society, *Cancer Response System*, No. 2,522, 23 Dec 1993

5 Jaffe, J.H., 'Drug addiction and drug abuse', in *The Pharmacological Basis of Therapeutics*, A.G. Gilman (ed), 6th edit. New York: Macmillan, 1980; US Surgeon General, *The Changing Cigarette*, Publication no. 81-51056, Washington, DC, Dept. of Health, Education and Welfare, 1981; Volle, R.L. and Koelle, G.B., 'Ganglionic stimulating and blocking agents', in Gilman, *op.cit.* 1975.

6 FDA report cited in *Los Angeles Times*, 18 July1994, p.A 12.

7 Palfai, T. and Jankiewicz, H., *Drugs and Human Behavior*, Dubuque, IA: Wm. C.

Brown, 1991.

8   Neiman, Richard, 'Aids and Smoking', *AIDS*, May 1993.

9   US Surgeon General, *The Health Consequences of Smoking*, Washington, DC: Government Printing Office, 1985.

10 Bulpitt C.J., Shipley M.J., Broughton P.M.G.,Fletcher A.E., Markowe H.L.J., Marmot M.G., 'The assessment of biological age', *Ageing Clin. Exp. Res.*, 1994, 6, pp.181–91.

11 Archives of Internal Medicine, Feb. 1993, reported in *University of California Wellness Letter*, 9 (8) May 1993, p.1.

12 American Cancer Society, *Cancer Response System*, 252, 1Sept 1992.

Chapter 11

1   Koob, G.F. and Weiss, F., 'Neuropharmacology of cocaine and ethanol dependence', *Recent Developments in Alcohol*, 10, 1992, pp.201-233

2   Miller, N.S. and Gold, M.S., 'A hypothesis for a common neurochemical basis for alcohol and drug disorders', *Psychiatric & Clinical Studies of North America*, 16 (1), March 1993, pp.105-17; see also: Witters, W. *et al*, *Drugs and Society*, Boston: Jones and Bartlett, 1992.

3   Morrisett, R.A. and Swartzwelder, H.S., in 'New insight may reduce alcohol impairment', *The Menninger Letter*, Aug. 1994, p.8, originally reported in *The Journal of Neuroscience*, 13(5).

4   McElduff, P and Dobson, AJ., 'How much alcohol and how often? Population based case-control study of alcohol consumption and risk of a major coronary event', *BMJ*, April 1997, 314, p.1159.

5   Russell, B., *The Conquest of Happiness*. New York: W.W. Norton, 1929. Revised 1996.

6   Dr Mary Dufour of the National Institute on Alcohol and Alcohol Abuse *Los Angeles Times*, 16 May 1994.

7   Maughan, R.J. et al., 'Factors influencing the restoration of fluid and electrolyte balance after exercise in the heat', British Journal of Sports Medicine, 31, 1997, 175–82.

8   Dimeff R.J., 'Steroids and other performance enhancers', in Matzen R.N. and Lang R.S., (eds), *Clinical Preventive Medicine*, St Louis: CV Mosby Co., 1993, p.367.

9   Affrime M.B., Lowenthal D.T., 'Effect of ethanol on metabolic responses to treadmill running in well-trained men', *J. Clin. Pharmacol.* 33, 1993, 136–9.

Chapter 12

1   Tumer N., LaRochelle J.S., Yurekli M., 'Exercise training reverses the age-related decline in tyrosine hydroxylase expression in rat hypothalamus', *J. Gerontol A. Biol. Sci. Med. Sci.*, 52 (5), Sept. 1997, pp.255–9.

2   Bam, J., *et al.*, 'Could women outrun men in ultramarathon races?', *Medical Science in Sports and Exercise*, 29 (2), 1997, pp.244–7.

3   Kushi, L.H., *Journal of American Medical Association.*, 277, 1997 pp.1287–92.

4   Klissouras, V., 'Aerobic power in old humans: genes and environment', World Congress of Sports Medicine, Orlando, FL, 31 May, 1998.

5   Blair, S.N., *et al.*, 'Influences of cardiorespiratory fitness and other precursors on cardiovascular disease and all-cause mortality in men and women', *Journal of the American Medical Association*, 276 (205–210), 1996.

6   Blair, S., 'Physical Activity, fitness and health: an overview', Presentation at the World Congress of Sports Medicine, Orlando, FL., 2 June 1998.

7   Morris, J.N., *et al.*, 'Exercise in leisure time', *British Heart Journal*, 63, 1990, pp 325–34.

8   Paffenbarger, R.S., *et al.*, 'Some interrelationships of physical activity, physiological fitness, health and longevity', in Bouchard, C., *et al.*, *Physical Activity in Fitness and Health*, Champaign, IL: Human Kinetics, 1993. p.119–33.

9   Kline, Porcari, Hintermeister, Freedson, Ward, McCarron, Ross and Rippe, 1987.

Chapter 13

1   Metter E.J., Conwit R., Tobin J., Fozard J.L., 'Age-associated loss of power and strength in the upper extremities in women and men', J. Gerontol A. Biol. Sci. Med. Sci., Sept.1997, pp. 267–76.

Chapter 14

1   Rider, R.A. and Daly, J. 'Effects of flexibility training on enhancing spinal mobility in older women', *Journal of Sports Medicine and Physical Fitness.* 31(2), June 1991, pp. 213–217.

Chapter 15

1   Ting, A., 'Running and the older athlete.' *Clinics in Sports Medicine.* 10 (2) April 1991, pp.319–325.

2   LeClercq, D., 'Ankle bracing in running: the effect of a push type medium ankle brace upon movements of the foot and ankle during the stance phase', *International Journal of Sports Medicine*, 18 (3) April 1997, pp. 222–228.

3   Swedenhag, J. and Seger, J., 'Running on land or in water: comparative exercise physiology.' *Medicine and Science in Sports and Exercise.* 24 (10), Oct. 1992, pp. 1,155–1,160.

4   Bergeron, M. et al., 'Fluid and Electrolyte losses during tennis in the heat'. Racquet Sports: *Clinics in Sports Medicine*, Vol 14,

1 Jan. 1995, W.B.Saunders: Philadelphia, 1995, p.23.

5   Pastene, J. *et al.*, 'Water balance during and after marathon running', *European Journal of Applied Physiology*, 73 (1 and 2), 1996, pp.49–55.

6   *See:* O'Connor, B. *et al.*, *Sports Injuries and Illnesses*, Marlborough, Wilts: Crowood Press, 1998. This book will give you the symptoms, treatment and prevention strategies for most sports-related injuries.

Chapter 16

1   Don Frankl, Paper delivered to the American Academy of Kinesiology, Washington, DC, April 1993.

2   Williams S. et al., 'Senior house officers' work related stressors, psychological distress, and confidence in performing clinical tasks in accident and emergency: a questionnaire study', *BMJ*, March 1997, 314, p.7,082 and 'Why workers suffer most from stress.' *Financial Times* , 26 Feb. 1995, *see* also *Healthy People 2000*, US Dept of Health and Human Services. Boston and London: Jones and Bartlett, 1990, p. 60.

3   Brunner, E., 'Socioeconomic determinants of health: Stress and the biology of inequality.' *BMJ.*, May, 1997, 314, p.1,472.

4   Kunst, A. et al., 'Occupational class and cause specific mortality in middle aged men in 11 European countries: comparison of population based studies', *BMJ*, 316, p.7,145.

5   Repetti, R.L., 'Short term effects of occupational stressors on daily mood and health complaints', *Health Psychology*, 112, 1993, pp.125131.

6   Herbert, J., 'Stress, the brain and mental illness', *BMJ*, Aug. 1997, 315, p.7,107.

7   Reported in Longevity, June 1993, p.60.

8   Harvard Women's Health Watch, Oct. 1994, p.6.

9   in *Stress Without Distress*, New York: Signet, 1975, p.83.

10 *Ibid.*, p.110.

11 Condensed from Spiegal, D., 'Ways to Cope with Life Threatening Illness' Quoted in *The Menninger Letter*, June 1994, p.4.

Chapter 17

1   Berger, Bonnie G., 'Coping with Stress: The effectiveness of exercise and other techniques', Paper presented at the Annual Meeting of the American Academy of Kinesiology and Physical Education, 24 March 1993. Published in *Quest*, 46, 1994.

2   Feuerstein, M., Labbe, E.E. and Kuczmierczyk, A.R., *Health Psychology: A Psychobiological Perspective*, New York: Plenum, 1986, p.189.

3   Dillbeck, M.C., Orme-Johnson, D.W., 'Physiological differences between transcendental meditation and rest', *American Psychologist*, 42, 1987, pp.879–81.

4   William Morrow: New York, 1975.

5   Berger, Bonnie, 'Mood Alteration with Exercise: A taxonomy to maximize benefits', Paper presented at the VIII World Congress of Sport Psychology, Lisbon, Portugal, 23 June 23 1993.

6   Boutcher, S.H. and Landers, D.M., 'The effects of vigorous exercise on anxiety, heart rate and alpha activity of runners and non-runners', *Psychophysiology*, 25, 1988, pp.696–702.

7   Raglin, J.S. and Morgan, W.P., 'Influences of exercise and quiet rest on state anxiety and blood pressure', *Medicine and Science in Sports and Exercise*, 19, 1987, pp.436–63.

8   Tucker, L.A., 'Effect of weight training on body attitudes: who benefits most?', *Journal of Sports Medicine and Physical Fitness*, 27, 1987, pp. 70–8; Young, M.L. 'Estimation of fitness and physical ability, physical performance, and self-concept among adolescent females', *Journal of Sports Medicine and Physical Fitness*, 25, 1985, pp.144–50.

9   Brown, J.D., 'Staying fit and staying well: physical fitness as a moderator of life stress', *Journal of Personality and Social Psychology*, 60, 1991, pp.555–61

10 Mackinnon, L.T., 'Exercise and immunology: current issues in exercise science', (Monograph No. 2), Champaign, IL: *Human Kinetics*, 1992; Sternfeld, B., 'Cancer and the protective effect of physical activity: the epidemiological evidence', *Medicine and Science in Sports and Exercise*, 24, 1991, pp.1195–209.

11 Berger, B.G., Friedman, E. and Easton, M., 'Comparison of jogging, the relaxation response, and group interaction for stress reduction', *Journal of Sport and Exercise Psychology*, 10, 1988, pp.431–47; Long, B.C. and Haney, C.J., 'Coping strategies for working women: Aerobic exercise and relaxation interventions', *Behavior Therapy*, 19, 1988, pp.75–83; Long and Haney, 'Long term follow up of stressed working women: a comparison of aerobic exercise and progressive relaxation', *Journal of Sport and Exercise Psychology*, 10, 1988, pp.461–70.

12 *The Menninger Letter*, June 1994, p.6.

Index